ॐ

YOGA

Surya Namaskar

Ashwini Kumar Aggarwal

जय गुरुदेव

ISBN13: 978-81-946198-3-3 Paperback Edition
ISBN13: 978-81-946198-4-0 Hardbound Edition
ISBN13: 978-81-946198-5-7 Digital Edition
ISBN13: 978-81-947338-9-8 B/W LowPrice Edition

Title: **YOGA Surya Namaskar**

Printed and Published by
Devotees of Sri Sri Ravi Shankar Ashram
34 Sunny Enclave, Devigarh Road,
Patiala 147001, Punjab, India

https://advaita56.weebly.com/
The Art of Living Centre

https://www.artofliving.org/

21st June 2020 Sunday, International Day of Yoga IDY 2020
Longest Day of the Year – Summer Solstice, Father's Day.
Annular Solar Eclipse – Amavasya, World Music Day.
Vikram Samvat 2077 Pramathi, Saka Era 1942 Sharvari

1st Edition June 2020

जय गुरुदेव

Dedication

Sri Sri Ravi Shankar

who gave us **Sun** Meditation
English https://www.youtube.com/watch?v=wXW2laakMLI
Hindi https://www.youtube.com/watch?v=Lc_uiVaLzqQ

an offering at thy lotus feet

Acknowledgements

An excellent online Sri Sri Yoga Level 1 course with bubbling participants and superlative faculty, 18-21 June 2020.

Content Creation Design Credits

Dipanshu Aggarwal Apurav Gupta Bubbling Satsang Group
Himika Sharma

Dipanshu17June2020 Shirsasana

https://www.youtube.com/watch?v=YpxstzvldQw

EEG signal based classification before and after combined Yoga and Sudarshan Kriya

https://www.sciencedirect.com/science/article/abs/pii/S0304394019303738

Blessing

Scientists say that the solar plexus is a storehouse of all your emotions. That's where you store your emotions, your gut feelings, all that is there. And it is of the size of small gooseberry, generally in everybody's system.

When you do Meditation it becomes the size of big lemon. That shows that you are emotionally stable and intuitively higher. Our ancient people have used this name Padmanabha, one whose navel has blossomed like a lotus.

Sri Sri Ravi Shankar

Bangalore Ashram, Satsang Dec 12, 2014

History of Surya Namaskar

Our Vedas eulogize the Sun, and there are many hymns in praise of the Surya Devata. Especially, the first chapter of the Krishna Yajur Veda Taittiriya Aranyakam has come to be known in recent times as the Surya Namaskar chapter.
http://vedicheritage.gov.in/aranyakas/taittiriya-aranyaka/

Taittiriya Aranyaka – South Indian Brahmins
https://en.wikipedia.org/wiki/Aranyaka

A hundred years ago in 1929, a book published by the Raja of Aundh named Surya Namaskars for Health, Efficiency & Longevity, marks the first official usage of this as a Yogic Asana Practice.

https://www.amazon.in/Surya-Namaskars-Ancient-Indian-Exercise-ebook/dp/B0827Y35WT
An excerpt
"One should strive to develop and strengthen the four principal parts of the body (Abdomen, Chest, Nervous System, & Excretory Organs), on the proper functioning of which all health depends. It has been found by actual experience that the SŪRYA NAMASKĀR exercise if regularly, methodically and scientifically done, renders these 4 parts fully developed and capable of resisting disease".

Contents

Prayer

ॐ भ॒द्रं कर्णे॑भिः शृणु॒याम॑ दे॒वाः । भ॒द्रं प॑श्ये मा॒क्षभि॒र् यज॑त्राः ।
स्थि॒रैरङ्गै॑स् तुष्टु॒वा(गुं)स॑स्त॒नूभिः॑ । व्यशे॑म दे॒वहि॑तं॒ यदायुः॑ ॥
स्व॒स्ति न॒ इन्द्रो॑ वृ॒द्धश्र॑वाः । स्व॒स्ति नः॑ पू॒षा वि॒श्ववे॑दाः ।
स्व॒स्ति न॒स्तार्क्ष्यो॒ अरि॑ष्टनेमिः । स्व॒स्ति नो॒ बृह॒स्पति॑र्दधातु ॥
ॐ शान्तिः॒ शान्तिः॒ शान्तिः॑ ॥

oṃ bhadraṃ karṇebhiḥ śṛṇuyāma devāḥ I bhadraṃ paśye
mākṣabhir yajatrāḥ I sthirairaṅgais tuṣṭuvā(guṃ)sastanūbhiḥ I
vyaśema devahitaṃ yadāyuḥ II svasti na indro vṛddhaśravāḥ I
svasti naḥ pūṣā viśvavedāḥ I svasti nastārkṣyo ariṣṭanemiḥ I
svasti no bṛhaspatirdadhātu II
oṃ śāntiḥ śāntiḥ śāntiḥ II

O Divine Light!
May our ears listen to the sacred and the auspicious.
May our eyes see the propitious allowing us
To come together to partake of wisdom.

May our limbs be firm and body attuned to long endurances.
May our senses function with full alertness and
May the sense of contentment be strong.

May our good thoughts form a discus to shield us and
May our education give us a shining personality.

Peace in our heart, in our body and in our environs.

http://vedicheritage.gov.in/Taittiriya_Aranyaka/KYTA_1.mp4

Bhagavad Gita

युक्ताहारविहारस्य , युक्तचेष्टस्य कर्मसु ।
युक्तस्वप्नावबोधस्य , योगो भवति दुःखहा ॥ ६.१७

yuktaahaaravihaarasya, yuktace.s.tasya karmasu |
yuktasvapnaavabodhasya, yogo bhavati du.hkhahaa || 6.17

6.17 Be regulated in food and exercise; be balanced in activity and duty. Take proper sleep and rest, and nurture senses equitably. Such a lifestyle leads to freedom from pain. It frees one from suffering. It extinguishes the pangs of remorse and banishes turmoil from life.

Regulated food includes eating fresh, vegetarian, timely meals . Regulated exercise includes Yogasana, walking, swimming, sports or gymnasium in a proper environment.

Balance in activity and duty includes having good teamwork, using the right tools, maintaining good posture and taking sufficient breaks for rest and hobby. Proper sleep includes using correct cot and mattress and sleeping with the lights off.

Nurturing senses equitably includes paying attention to brushing twice daily, taking care of hair and skin by appropriate massage, taking care of eyes and ears and ensuring correct breathing.

What is Surya Namaskar

Surya Namaskar is a fundamental set of 12 postures to step into a higher state of consciousness that reflects Purity.

It leads to Yoga, or the significant moment when one relaxes, absorbed in divine union.

The entire process comprises of

- A Cheerful beginning
- Stepping onto the Yogamat facing EAST
- Having a sip of Water to begin with
- Chanting Om Suryaaya Namah

This entire process is another name for creating your own Wonderful Day.

It is a proven cardiovascular workout of a high order, when done at a smooth pace.

When done with holding the stretch at each pose with normal breathing, it is meditative, relaxing and toning.

The Sun is traditionally connected to the Manipura Chakra, known as the Navel Center, or the Solar Plexus. It is also the 2nd brain of the body, where all the nerves meet, and the place of the umbilical cord connecting every new born.

We see that all the poses in the Surya Namaskar have a significant effect on the solar plexus. In other words these asanas massage, strengthen, realign, and invigorate the gut. That by default in medical parlance is the prime source of illness prevention and cure.

So both physically and spiritually, the Sun Salutation set of poses has a profound impact.

Source of Sun Salutation Mantras

Bhanu Saptami Shloka (Excerpts) invoking the Sun

आदित्य–नमस्कारान् ये कुर्वन्ति दिने दिने । One who salutes the Orb daily,
दीर्घ आयुर्–बलं वीर्य तेजस् तेषां च जायते । Long Life, Strength, Vigor, Luster all in him get infused,
अकाल–मृत्यु–हरणं सर्व–व्याधि–विनाशनम् । Untimely death is prevented, all illnesses are banished,
सूर्य–पादोदकं तीर्थं जठरे धारयामि अहम् ॥ Water that flows over the shining feet, that nectar in my belly I entertain.
॥ ॐ श्री सवितृ–सूर्य–नारायणाय नमः ॥ Prostrations to the one who purifies the intellect, makes reason resplendent all-encompassing, and he who pervades the entire creation.

Aditya Hridayam Stotra (Excerpts) glorifying the Sun

आदित्यः[9] सविता[10] सूर्यः[3] खगः[5] पूषा[6] गभस्तिमान् ।
सुवर्णसदृशो भानु[4]र्हिरण्यरेता दिवाकरः ॥ १०
हरिदश्वः सहस्रार्चिः सप्तसप्तिर्मरीचि[8]मान् ।
तिमिरोन्मथनः शम्भुस्त्वष्टा मार्ताण्ड अंशुमान् ॥ ११
हिरण्यगर्भः[7] शिशिरस्तपनो भास्करो[12] रविः[2] ।
अग्निगर्भोऽदितेः पुत्रः शङ्खः शिशिरनाशनः ॥ १२
व्योमनाथस्तमोभेदी ऋग्यजुःसामपारगः ।
घनवृष्टिरपां मित्रो[1] विन्ध्यवीथीप्लवङ्गमः ॥ १३
आतपी मण्डली मृत्युः पिङ्गलः सर्वतापनः ।
कवि[11]र्विश्वो महातेजाः रक्तः सर्वभवोद्भवः ॥ १४ (note – कवि means अर्क)
नक्षत्रग्रहताराणामधिपो विश्वभावनः ।
तेजसामपि तेजस्वी द्वादशात्मन् नमोऽस्तु ते ॥ १५
Salutations to the 12 glorious forms and virtues of the Sun.

The 12 Mantras

This is the ultimate aim of yoga practice.
To be sensitive, sensible, available. To exude love and compassion.
To care for nature, to serve humanity, and
to be full of laughter and peace.

<table>
<tr><td rowspan="2">1</td><td>Om Mitrāya Namaḥ</td><td>ॐ मित्राय नमः (मित्र)</td></tr>
<tr><td colspan="2">Adoration to a dear friend</td></tr>
<tr><td rowspan="2">2</td><td>Om Ravaye Namaḥ</td><td>ॐ रवये नमः (रवि)</td></tr>
<tr><td colspan="2">Adoration to he who guides positive transformation</td></tr>
<tr><td rowspan="2">3</td><td>Om Suryāye Namaḥ</td><td>ॐ सूर्याय नमः (सूर्य)</td></tr>
<tr><td colspan="2">Adoration to the one who activates and spurs forward</td></tr>
<tr><td rowspan="2">4</td><td>Om Bhānave Namaḥ</td><td>ॐ भानवे नमः (भानु)</td></tr>
<tr><td colspan="2">Adoration to the luminous one</td></tr>
<tr><td rowspan="2">5</td><td>Om Khagāya Namaḥ</td><td>ॐ खगाय नमः (खग)</td></tr>
<tr><td colspan="2">Adoration to he who does space travel</td></tr>
<tr><td rowspan="2">6</td><td>Om Pūṣṇe Namaḥ</td><td>ॐ पूष्णे नमः (पूषन्)</td></tr>
<tr><td colspan="2">Adoration to the nourisher of all</td></tr>
<tr><td rowspan="2">7</td><td>Om Hiranyagarbhāya Namaḥ</td><td>ॐ हिरण्यगर्भाय नमः</td></tr>
<tr><td colspan="2">Adoration to the golden womb</td></tr>
<tr><td rowspan="2">8</td><td>Om Marīchye Namaḥ</td><td>ॐ मरीचये नमः (मरीचि)</td></tr>
<tr><td colspan="2">Adoration to the one full of effulgent rays</td></tr>
<tr><td rowspan="2">9</td><td>Om Ādityāya Namaḥ</td><td>ॐ आदित्याय नमः (आदित्य)</td></tr>
<tr><td colspan="2">Adoration to he who is first born with Time and Space</td></tr>
<tr><td rowspan="2">10</td><td>Om Savitre Namaḥ</td><td>ॐ सवित्रे नमः (सवितृ))</td></tr>
<tr><td colspan="2">Adoration to he who purifies the intellect</td></tr>
<tr><td rowspan="2">11</td><td>Om Arkāya Namaḥ</td><td>ॐ अर्काय नमः (अर्क)</td></tr>
<tr><td colspan="2">Adoration to the one worthy of glory</td></tr>
<tr><td rowspan="2">12</td><td>Om Bhāskarāya Namaḥ</td><td>ॐ भास्कराय नमः</td></tr>
<tr><td colspan="2">Adoration to he who dispels ignorance</td></tr>
</table>

https://yogainternational.com/article/view/sun-salutations-with-mantras
https://www.youtube.com/watch?v=TcLVgwKRvKA

The 12 Asanas

1	Prayer Pose प्रणाम आसन	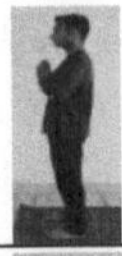	NAMASTE
2	Raised Arms Pose हस्त उत्तान आसन	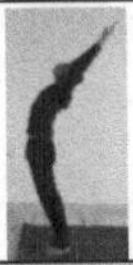	UP & BACK
3	Hands to Feet Pose हस्त पाद् आसन	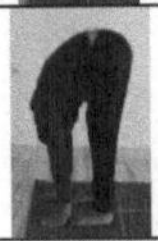	Forward & DOWN
4	Horse Rider Pose अश्व सञ्चालन आसन	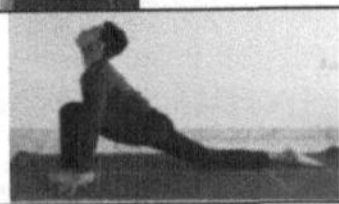	RIGHT LEG BACK
5	Plank Pose चतुरङ्ग दण्ड आसन	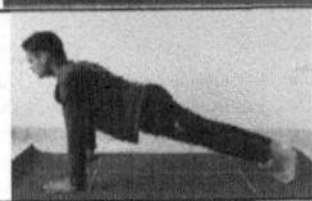	OTHER LEG BACK
6	Prostration Pose अष्टाङ्ग नमस्कार	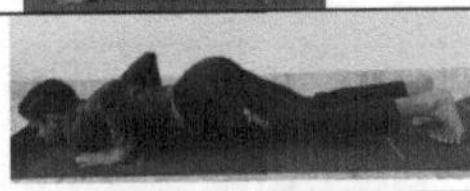	ASHTANGA PRANAAM
7	Cobra Pose भुजङ्ग आसन	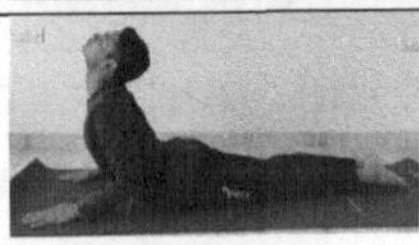	BHUJANGASANA
8	Downward Facing Dog अधो मुख श्वान आसन	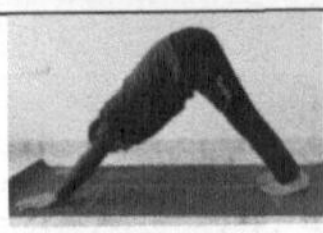	DOWNWARD DOG
9	Horse Rider Pose अश्व सञ्चालन आसन	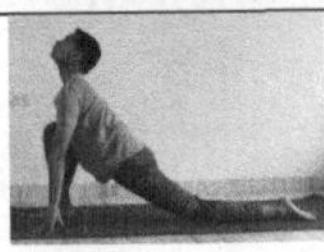	RIGHT LEG FRONT
10	Hands to Feet Pose हस्त पाद् आसन	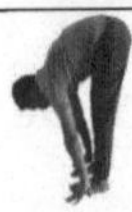	OTHER LEG FRONT
11	Raised Arms Pose हस्त उत्तान आसन	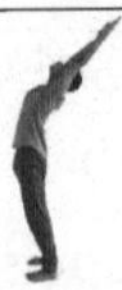	UP & BACK
12	Prayer Pose प्रणाम आसन	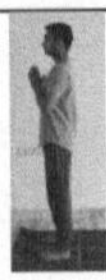	NAMASTE

The 12 Sets

Technically, 2 rounds of Surya Namaskar make 1 set.

24 rounds of Surya Namaskar make 12 sets. With alternate leg going back and front during each round.

108 rounds of Surya Namaskar are 54 sets. The ideal. It takes 40 minutes done at a smooth pace.

Yogathon Count 108
https://www.youtube.com/watch?v=ai59VYzouFE

Nature of the Body

Body enjoys hard work. Good physical labor thrills the body.

Routine and similar simple activity brings out the best in the body, which then steadily grows in strength day by day.

Patanjali Yoga Sutras

स्थिरसुखमासनम् ॥ २.४६ ॥ sthirasukhamāsanam ॥ 2.46 ॥

स्थिर-सुखम् आसनम् ।

2.46 Asana is that which is Stable and Comfortable

Gheranda Samhita

आसनानि समस्तानि यावन्तो जीवजन्तवः ।

चतुरशीति-लक्षाणि शिवेन कथितानि च ॥ २.१

2.1 Body Postures or Asanas are as many as there are species of insects, birds, and animals. This has been stated by the all-knowing great Lord and attested by the soul's travel through various bodies before attaining a human birth.

Nature of the Mind

Mind loves new stuff. Mind wants excitement, show off and Complexity. It is a superhuman task to baby-sit, cajole, and step-by-step culture the mind.

One will definitely benefit from being in the company of the Wise. Attending discourses and having satsang with the Saints. Especially when one surrenders to a Master, then the Guru assumes the responsibility of our mind to a sufficient degree.

> Patanjali Yoga Sutras
> **योगश्चित्तवृत्तिनिरोधः** ॥ १.२ ॥ yogaścittavr̥ttinirodhaḥ । 1.2
>
> योगः चित्त–वृत्ति–निरोधः ।
> Yogic Life entails a Calming of the Processes in the Mind

Proper Breathing

Breath is the veritable link between the body and the mind. When we are agitated or angry, our breath has a noticeable pulsation, and when we are relaxed and happy, our breath is soft and unnoticeable.

Conversely, it is an established fact that changing the breathing pattern changes the thoughts in the mind, and has a profound effect on the body as well.

The famous Sudarshan Kriya powerful breathing technique taught in the Art of Living Happiness courses worldwide is a proven testimony and an established remedy for culturing the mind and strengthening the body by means of the Breath.

Gheranda Samhita

अथातः सम्प्रवक्ष्यामि प्राणायामस्य सद्विधिम् ।

यस्य साधनमात्रेण देवतुल्यो भवेत् नरः ॥ ५.१

athātaḥ sampravakṣyāmi prāṇāyāmasya sadvidhim I

yasya sādhanamātreṇa devatulyo bhavet naraḥ II 5.1

5.1 Now in proper and precise detail hear from me the correct method of Breath control Pranayama. Its judicious practice makes a human akin to the celestials in virtues, splendor and vitality.

Proper Diet

No progress is possible if our diet is mainly fast food, on the run, and without a plan.

> Gheranda Samhita
>
> शुद्धं सु–मधुरं स्निग्धम् उदर–अर्ध–विवर्जितम् ।
>
> भुज्यते सु–रसं प्रीत्या मित–आहारम् इमं विदुः ॥ ५.२१
>
> śuddhaṃ su–madhuraṃ snigdham udara–ardha–vivarjitam I
>
> bhujyate su–rasaṃ prītyā mita–āhāram imaṃ viduḥ II 5.21
>
> 5.21 Pure and Freshly prepared,
> delicious,
> good for the nerves and muscles,
> half-belly full
>
> Nourishing to the soul,
> inclusive of juices and soups and well cooked,
> such is the diet friendly to the body and mind.

What to Eat, Diet Plan - Sadhguru
https://www.youtube.com/watch?v=yQjtZrwdPjY

Diet is not just intake through the mouth. Whatever we take in through every sense is the DIET and it modulates the MIND.

5 Tips to Naturally Cleanse Your Body at Home – Sadhguru
https://www.youtube.com/watch?v=6_eZjroYURU

Warm Ups

It is a good practice to warm up a bit by a walk, light jog, or simply moving the joints of the neck, shoulder, and ankle a few times.

A very good pelvic opener, thighs, hips, and knees relaxer is the Butterfly Dynamic Pose.

For massaging the Spine, try the Cat Stretch Dynamic Pose.

A quick and easy whole body loosener is the Bridge Pose.

Making Rain with the Arms n Palms
Blinking the Eyes
Massaging the Ears
Take good care of yourself
REGULARLY

BRIDGE

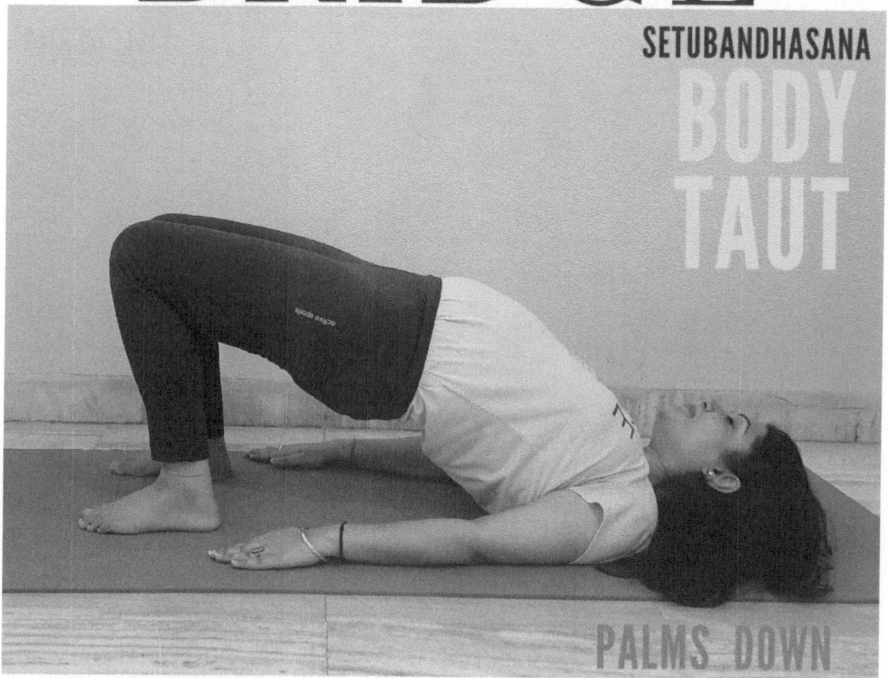

A nice lift of the torso in a gentle sloping arch. Feet firmly planted.

Elbows Straight. Shoulders anchored

NECK FIRM

Maintain focus on lumbar low back, make each breath smooth s l o w quiver-free

POSE FOR 6 BREATHS

BUTTERFLY

TITLI ASANA

BODY

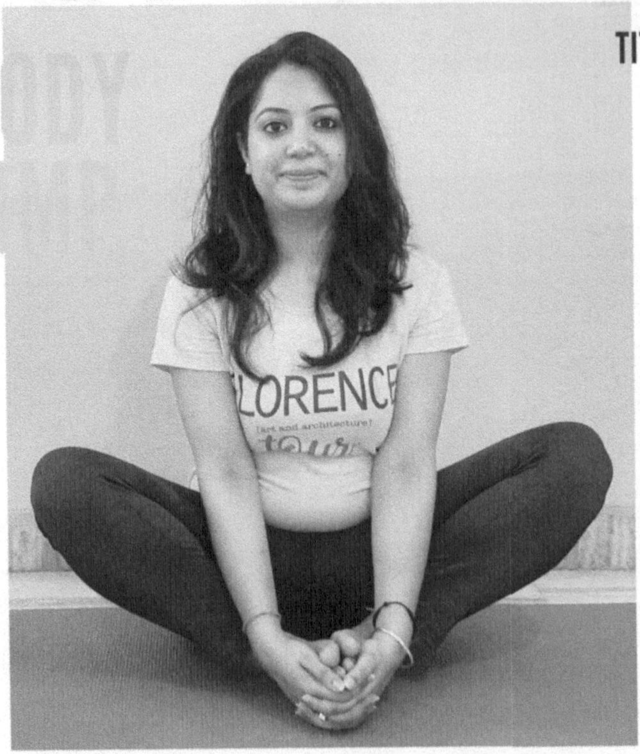

FLAP THE LEGS MIMIC A BUTTERFLY

FLY CHEERFULLY FOR 2 MINUTES

BUTTERFLY

TITLI ASANA

BODY LIMP

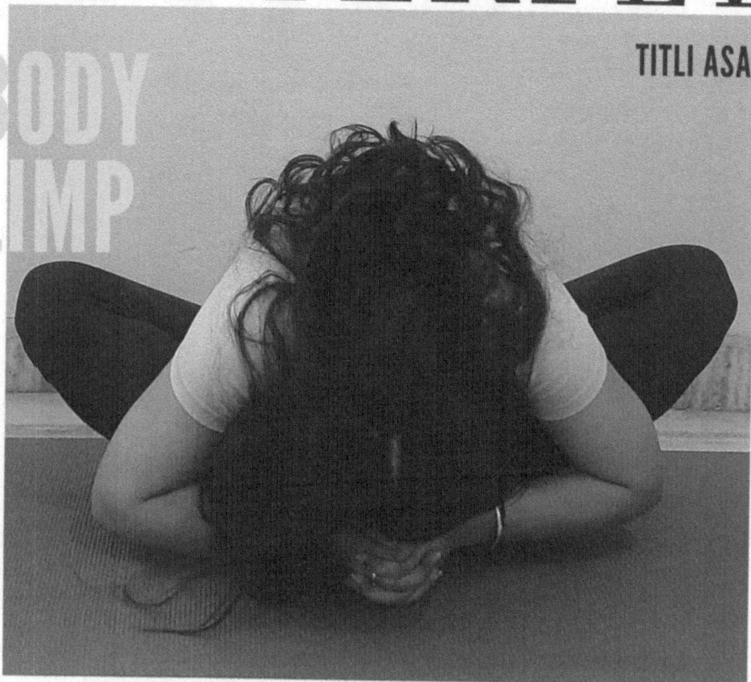

AFTER BUTTERFLYING BOW DOWN

BOW FOR FEW SECONDS

CAT

MARJARIASANA

BODY LIMP

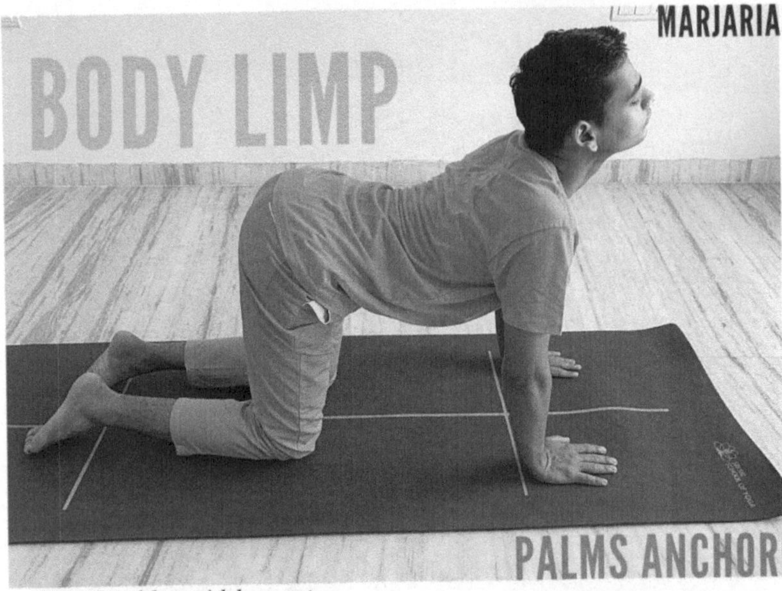

PALMS ANCHORED

Feet shoulder width apart. Knees supported on Mat. Lift up to Table pose.

Breathe In Spine goes down Head comes up.

SPINE MOVES

Maintain focus on Spine, make each breath smooth s l o w quiver-free

POSE FOR 6 BREATHS

Before Beginning

Some preparations done beforehand deepen the satisfaction and make it rewarding.

Pleasantly Lit, Well Ventilated Room

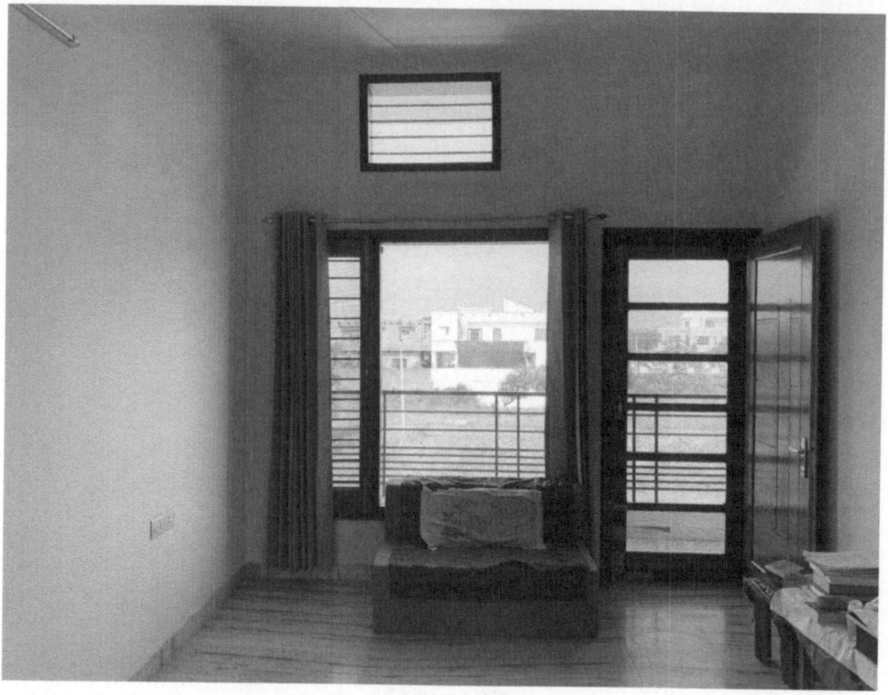

Yoga Mat and Water Bottle

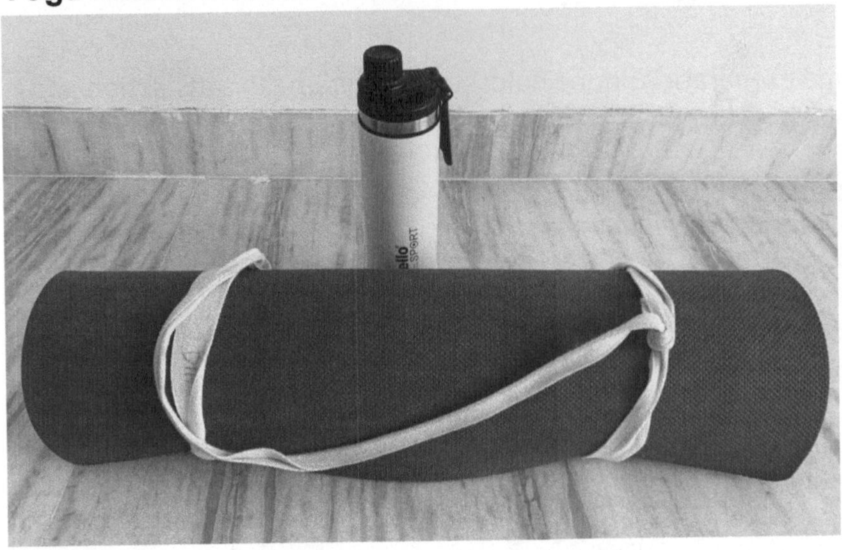

Begin with a Gratefulness

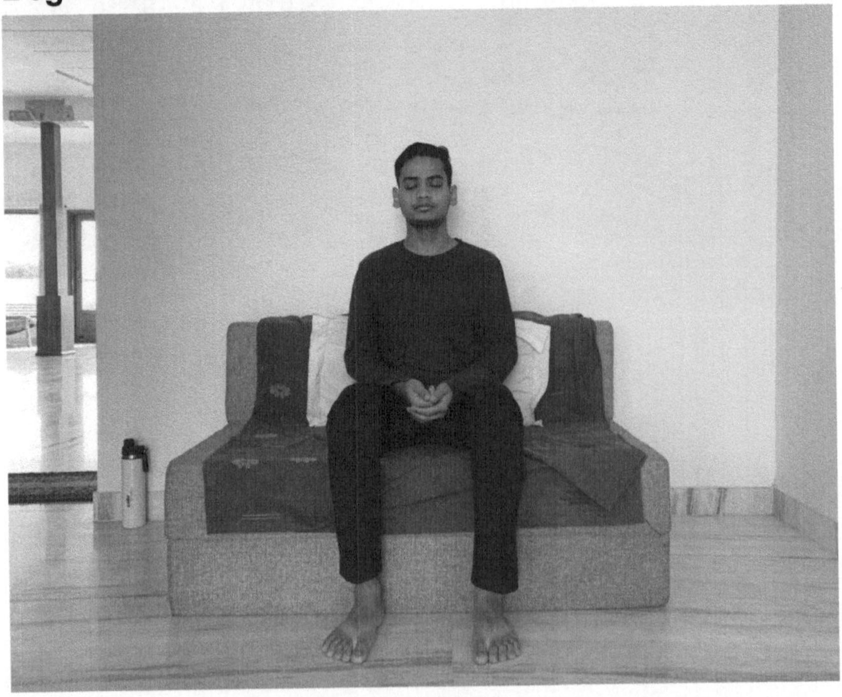

Sun Salutation Practice

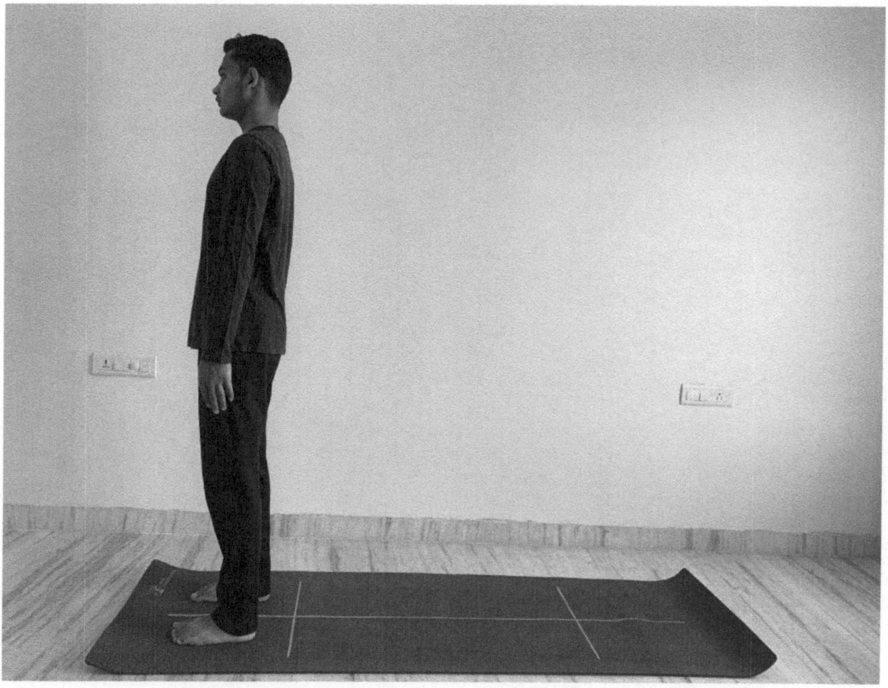

Step to the front of your Yogamat.
Be relaxed with hands loosely by the sides.
Feet comfortable distance apart.

Take a moment to be with yourself.

Stand Steady, Stand Tall, Be Yourself. It will take some practice to become still and it is not at all as easy as it sounds. This pose makes many changes in the physiology as one comes to grips with oneself. It is a variation of Tadasana.

One needs to become aware of one's anatomy and if there is any strain or stiffness anywhere. One needs to see if one can hold the pose with gentle deep breathing, or if the breath is erratic. One needs to observe if the thoughts are racing...

01 Namaste – Pranaam Asana

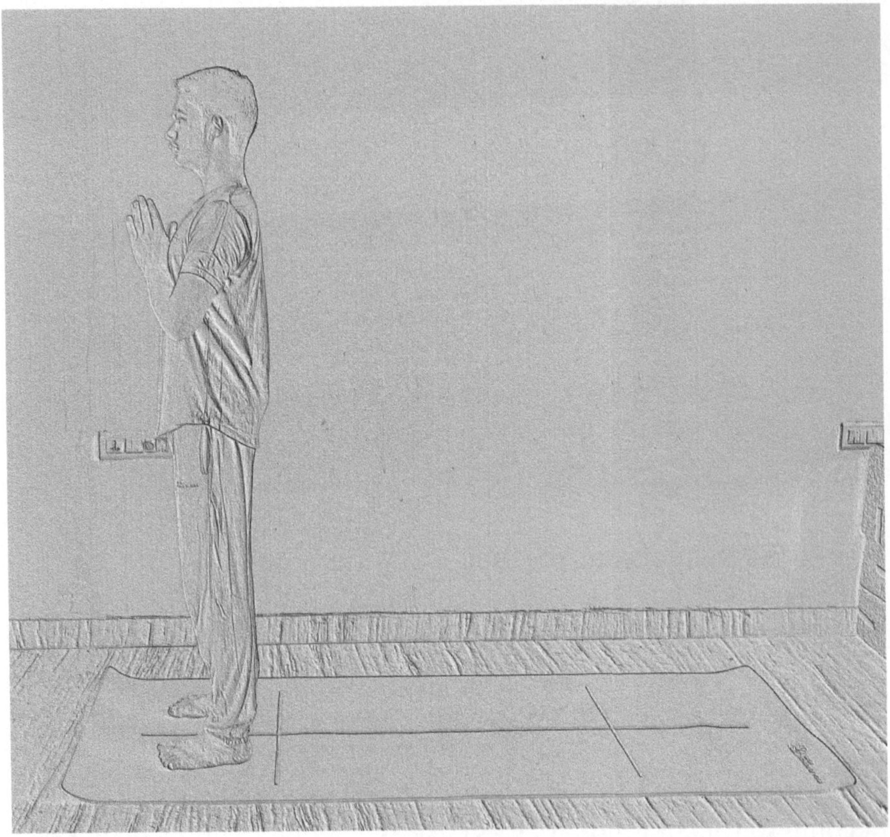

01 Namaste

Our YOGA Practice is so Beautifully Designed. We begin with a prayer that is so natural and graceful. We take a moment to honor the creation and honor ourself.

Seeing Purity Within and Without.
Opens our Mind to the Infinite.

Ensure that POCKETS are EMPTY. Clothes are Loose, yet Elegant.

If convenient, FACE towards EAST.

Walk up to the top of your Yoga Mat.

- Stand Feet Apart. Shoulders Relaxed. Head Straight.
- Breathe IN, bring both arms UP from the sides.
- Join the palms at chest level.
- Observe the ambience and observe the silence.
- Allow the breath to become slow and deep.
- May bend forward just a bit in reverence. Or simply feel it in the heart.

Either
We chant the various mantras at each pose, or
We chant Om Suryāya Namaḥ at pose 1 and then go on for the remaining poses silently, or
We do it all in silence without any mantra or japa.

NAMASTE

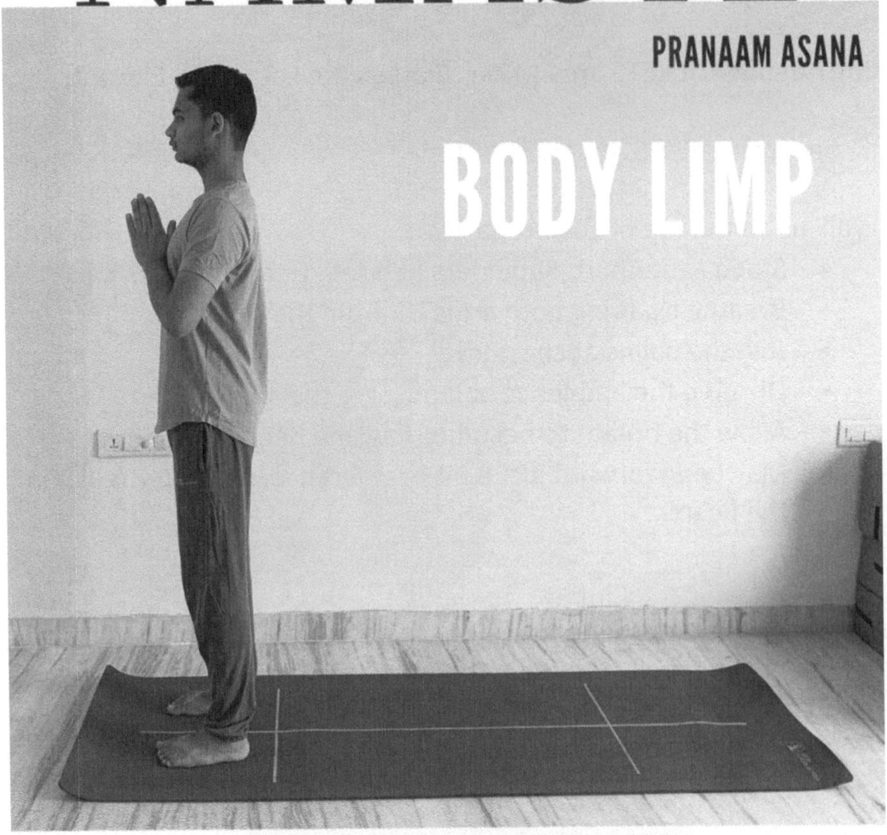

I AM THE MOST FORTUNATE
CREATION LOVES ME

NAMASTE

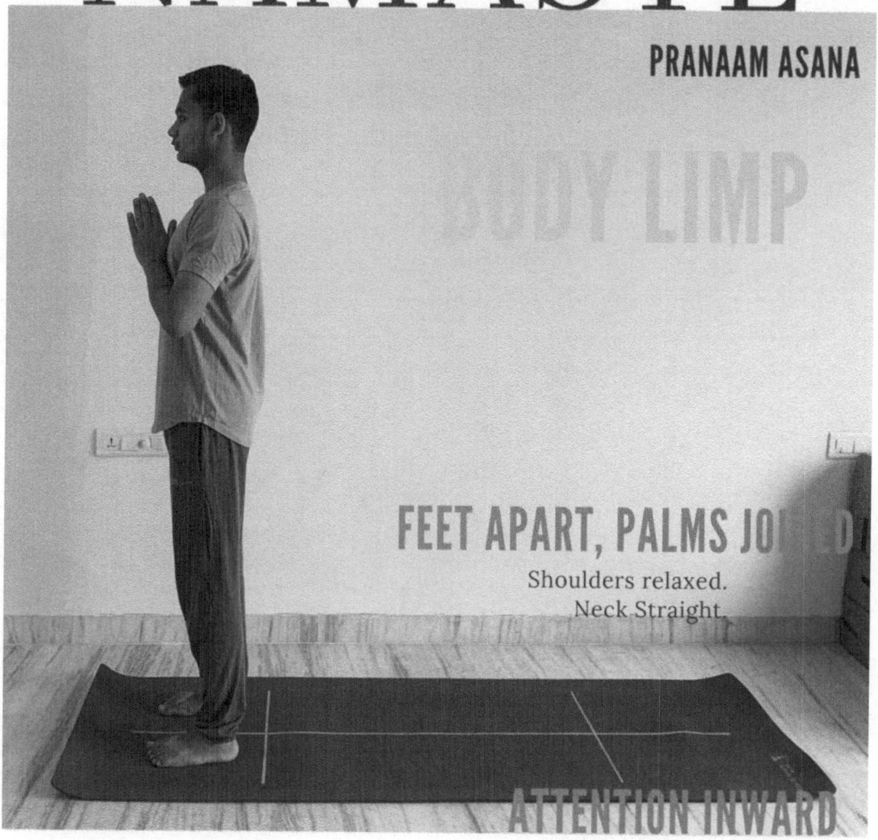
PRANAAM ASANA
BODY LIMP
FEET APART, PALMS
Shoulders relaxed.
Neck Straight.
ATTENTION INWARD

Maintain focus on Grace
received, make each breath
smooth s l o w quiver-free

POSE FOR 2 BREATHS

02 Up and Back – Hasta Uttana Asana

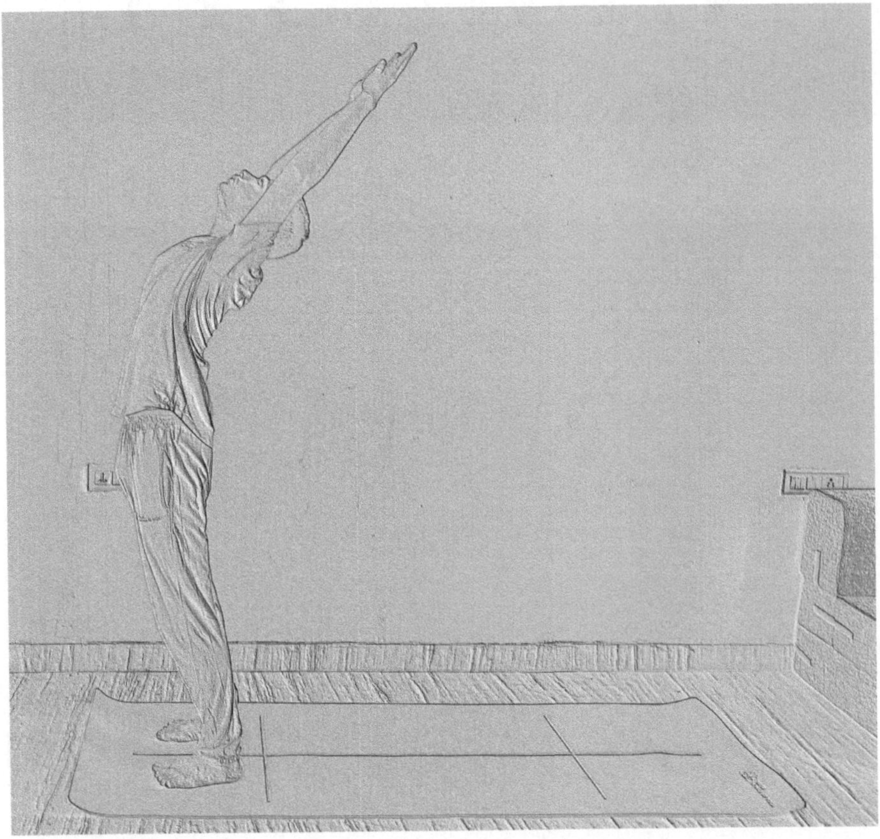

02 Up and Back

Without shifting the Feet from Pose 1

- Breathe IN, raise both arms over the head.
- Go back.
- Open the chest, bend slightly from the waist.
- Look up to the ceiling or
  the mild Sun in the early morning dawn Sky.
- Observe the ambience and observe the silence.
- Allow the breath to become slow and deep.

UP & BACK

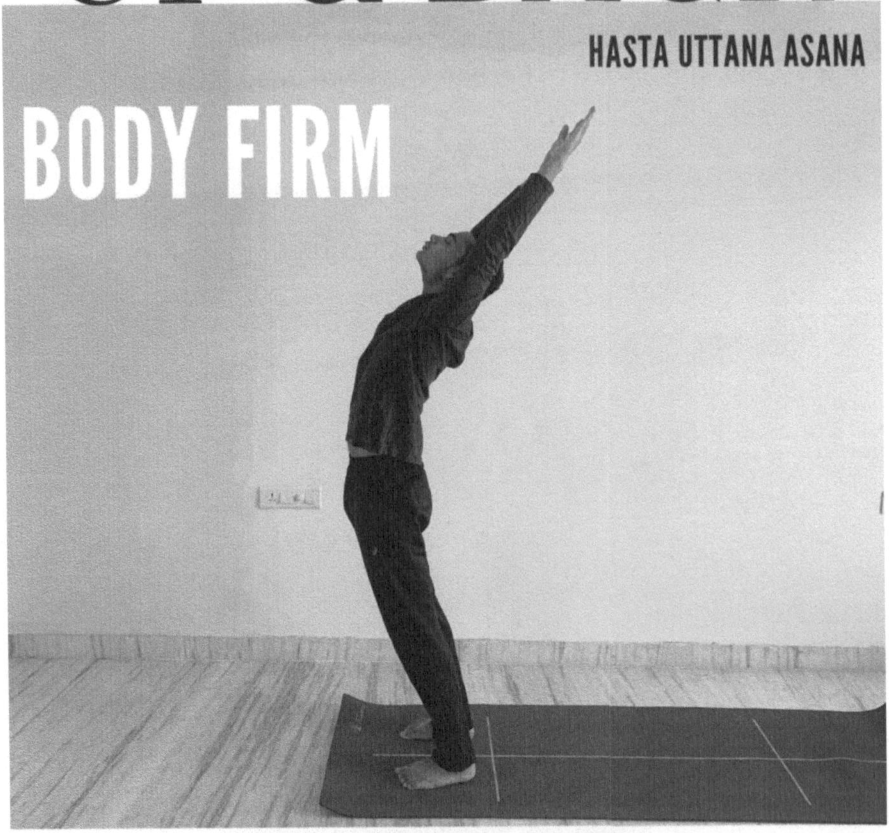

GENTLE ARCHING BEAUTY
BUILDS CONFIDENCE

UP & BACK

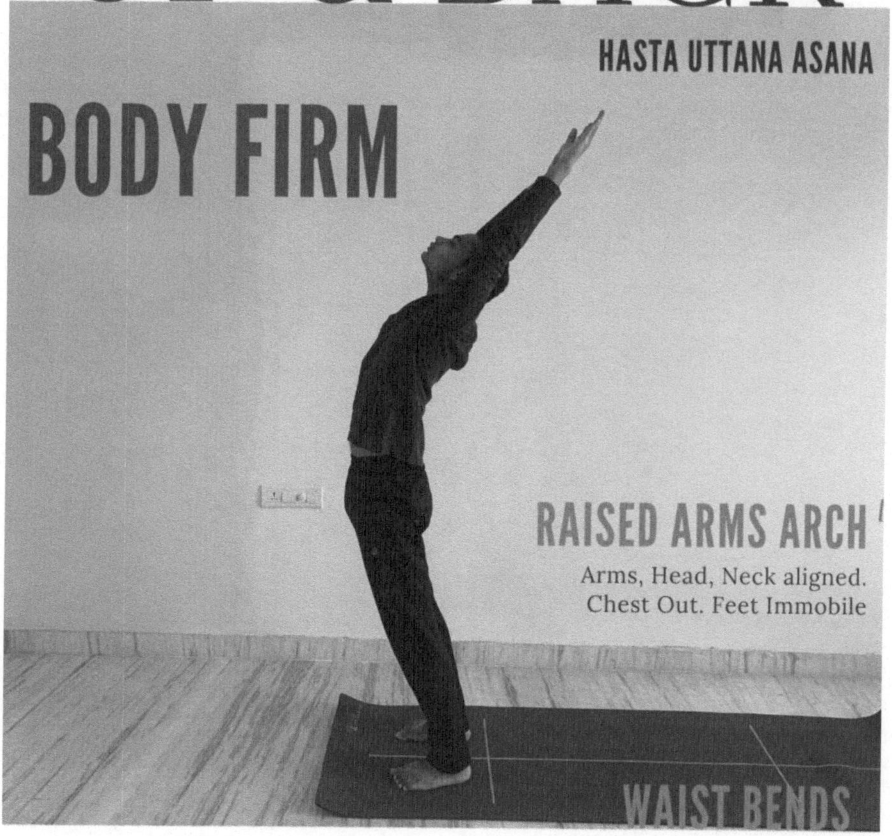
HASTA UTTANA ASANA
BODY FIRM
RAISED ARMS ARCH
Arms, Head, Neck aligned.
Chest Out. Feet Immobile
WAIST BENDS

Maintain focus on Waist,
make each breath smooth
s l o w quiver-free

POSE FOR 2 BREATHS

03 Forward and Down – Hasta Pada Asana

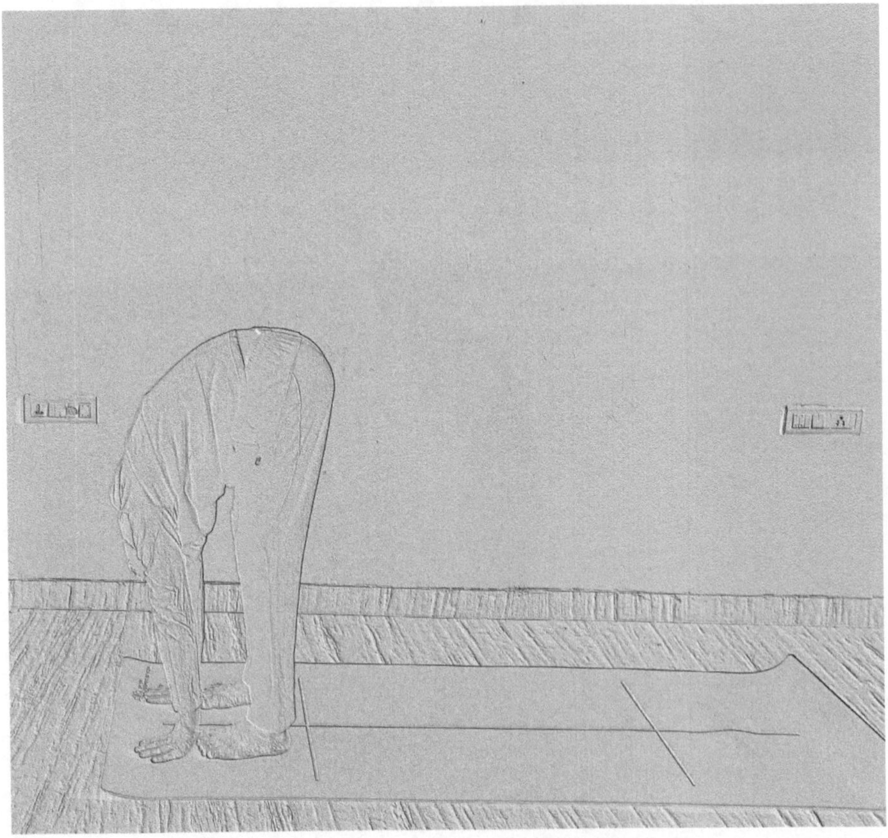

03 Forward Bend

Without shifting the Feet from Pose 2

- Breathe OUT, slowly lower both arms.
- Go Forward from the Waist.
- Keep the Head in between both Arms
- Go all the way till the palms touch the floor
- Ensure that Knees are straight.
- Allow the shoulders arms to be relaxed while maintaining taut the knees.
- Observe the ambience and observe the silence.
- Allow the breath to become slow and deep.

AND DOWN

FORWARD

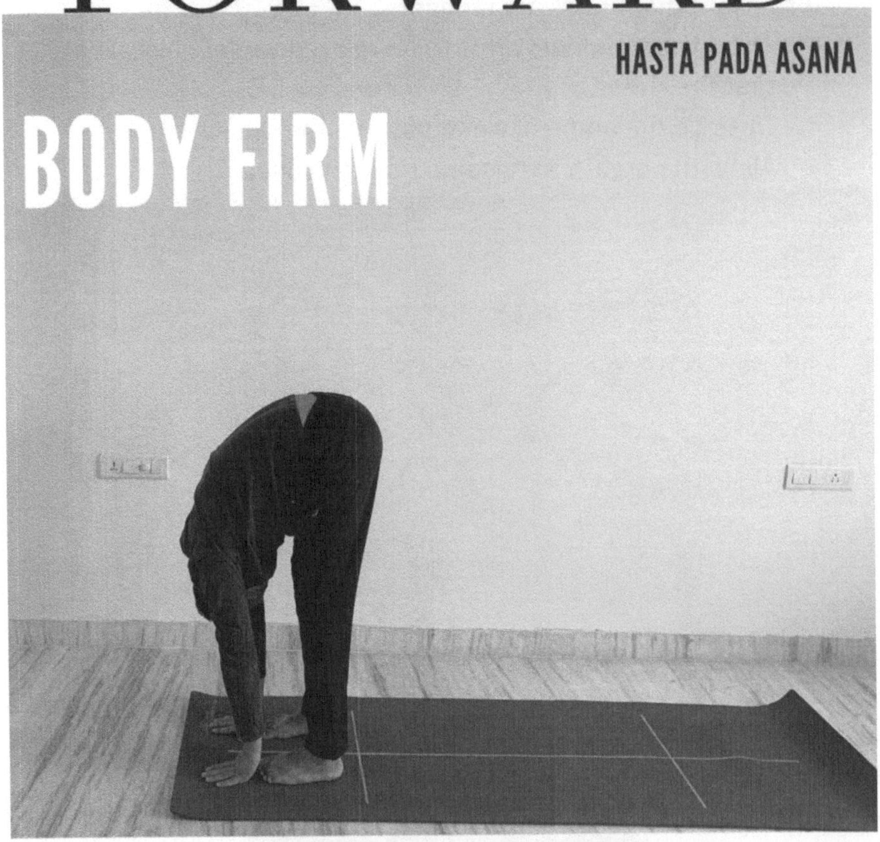

UNDER KNEE PRESSURE
KEEPS KNEE FLUIDS INTACT

AND DOWN

FORWARD

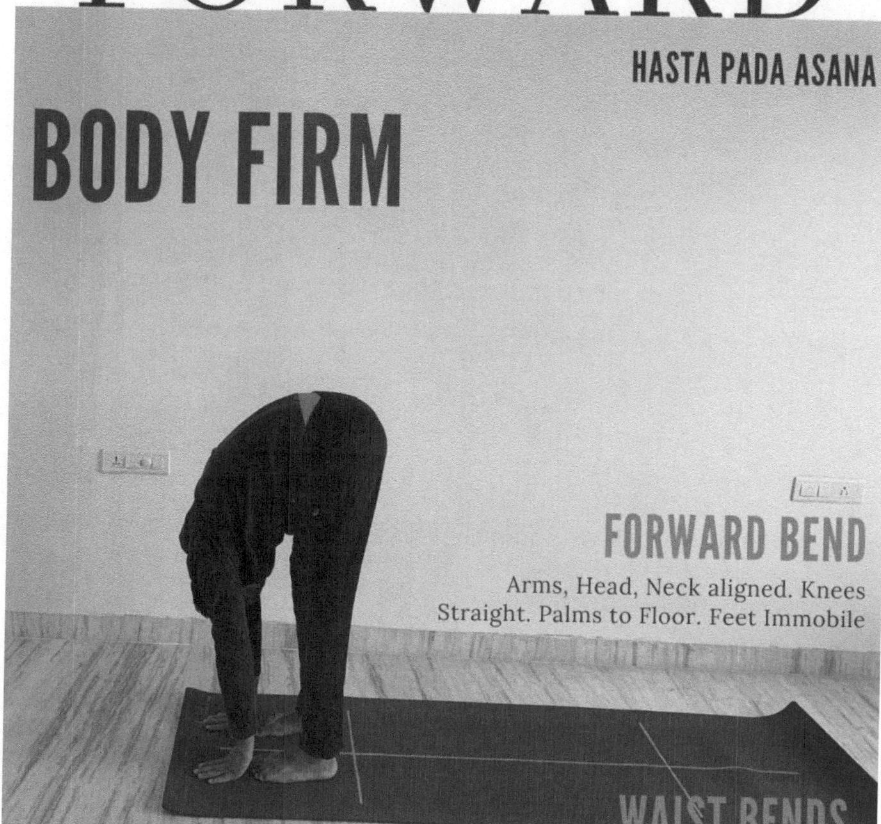
HASTA PADA ASANA
BODY FIRM
FORWARD BEND
Arms, Head, Neck aligned. Knees Straight. Palms to Floor. Feet Immobile
WAIST BENDS

Maintain focus on Knees,
make each breath smooth
s l o w quiver-free

POSE FOR 2 BREATHS

04 Right Leg Back – Ashva Sanchalana Asana

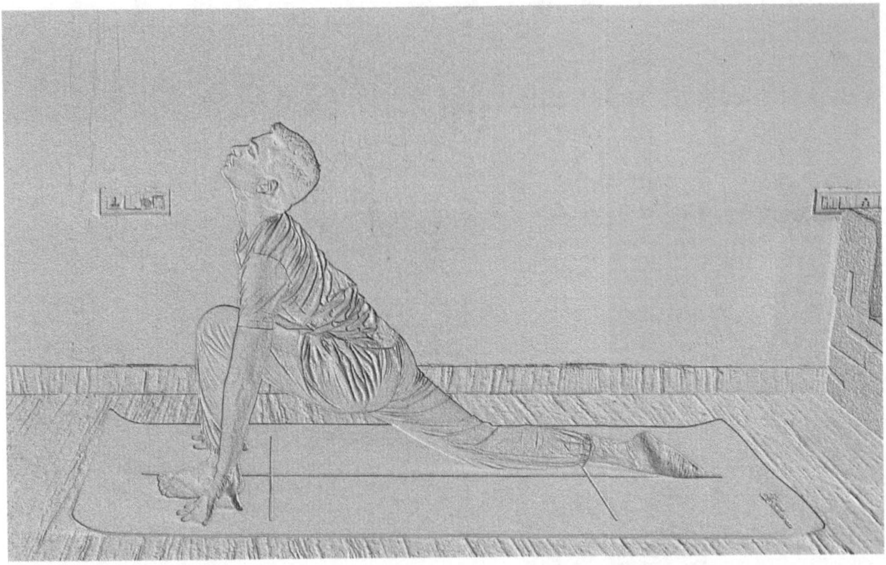

04 Right Leg Back

Without shifting the Feet from Pose 3

- Bend the knees to place both palms besides the feet on the outside.
- With palms firmly anchored on the floor,
- Keep the left leg where it was immobile.
- Take the Right Leg back all the way.
- Allow the Right knee to touch the floor
- Open the Right foot to lie on the floor.
- Now tilt the head back, look up towards the ceiling or the mild Sun in the early morning dawn Sky.
- Observe the ambience and observe the silence.
- Allow the breath to become slow and deep.

BACK

RIGHT LEG

ASHVA SANCHALANA ASANA

BODY FIRM

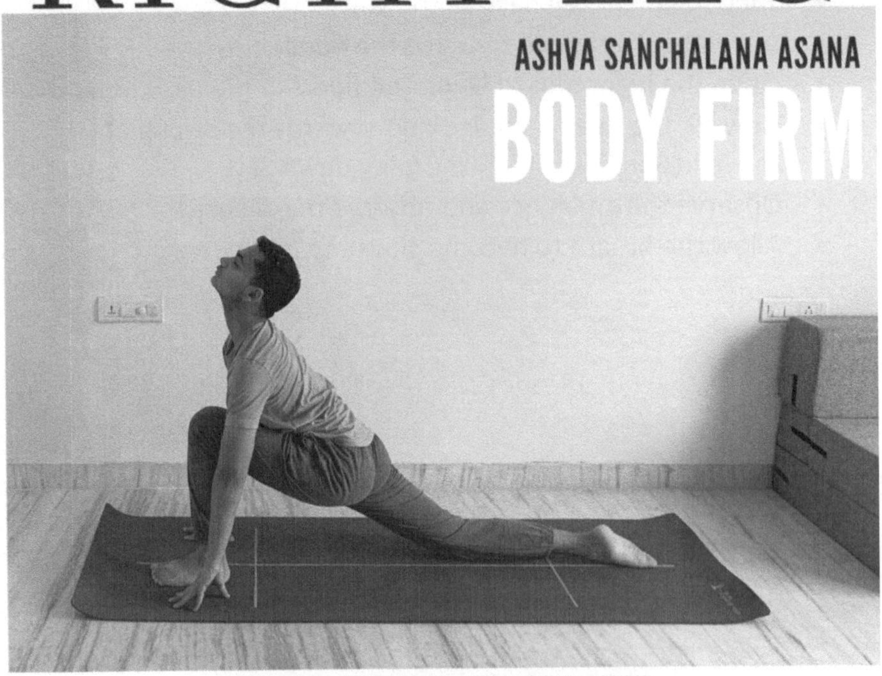

HORSE RIDING IS THE KEY
ALL ANCESTORS RODE THEM

POSE FOR 2 BREATHS

RIGHT LEG BACK

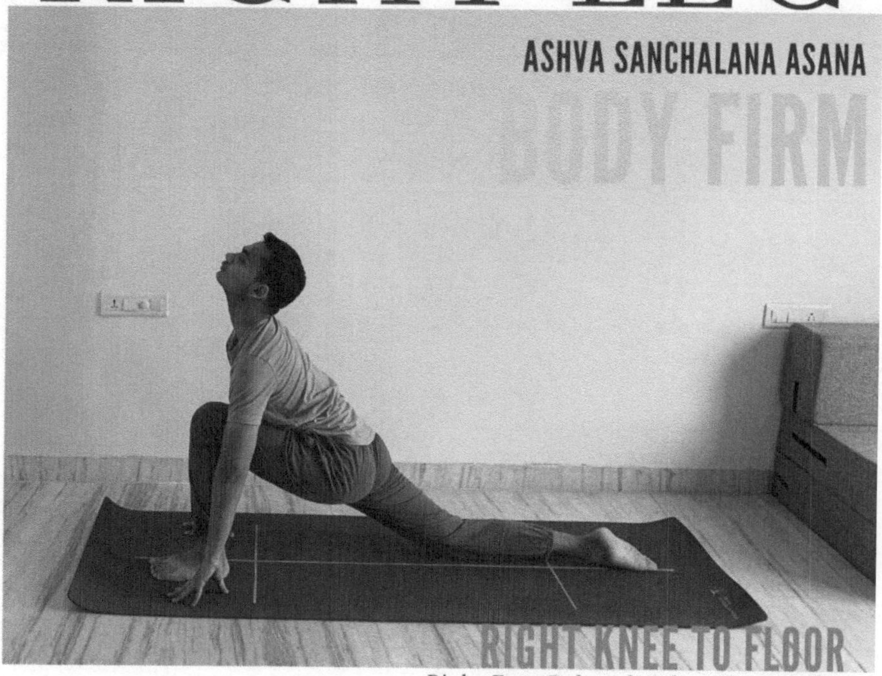

Right Foot Relaxed. A fine Horse Rider Balance.

HEAD TILTED BACK

Maintain focus on Balance, make each breath smooth s l o w quiver-free

POSE FOR 2 BREATHS

05 Left Leg Back – Chaturanga Danda Asana

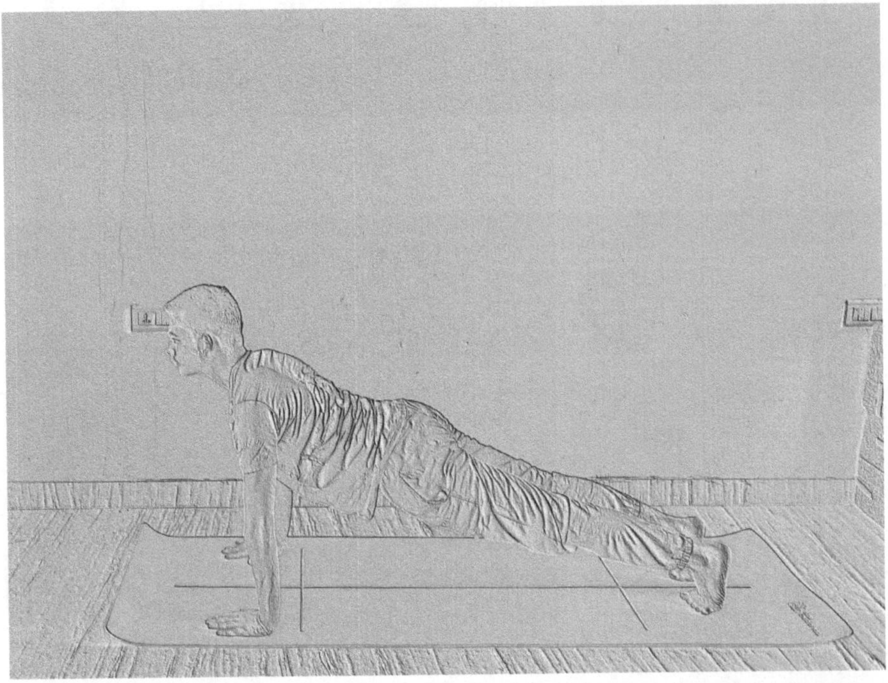

05 Left Leg Back as well

Without shifting the palms from Pose 4

- Take the Left Leg back all the way.
- Make the entire torso in one line
- Ensure the knees are straight
- Come up on your toes, palms anchored as before
- Observe the ambience and observe the silence.
- Allow the breath to become slow and deep.

PLANK

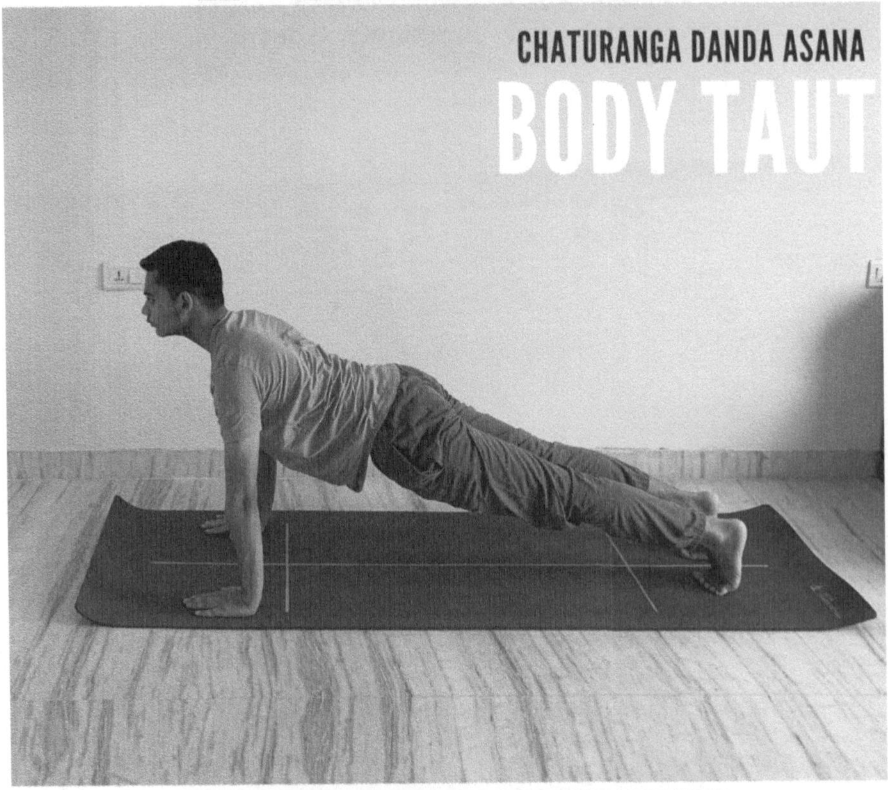

STRAIGHT PLANKS MAKE HOMES & ANATOMY WELL

POSE FOR 2 BREATHS

PLANK

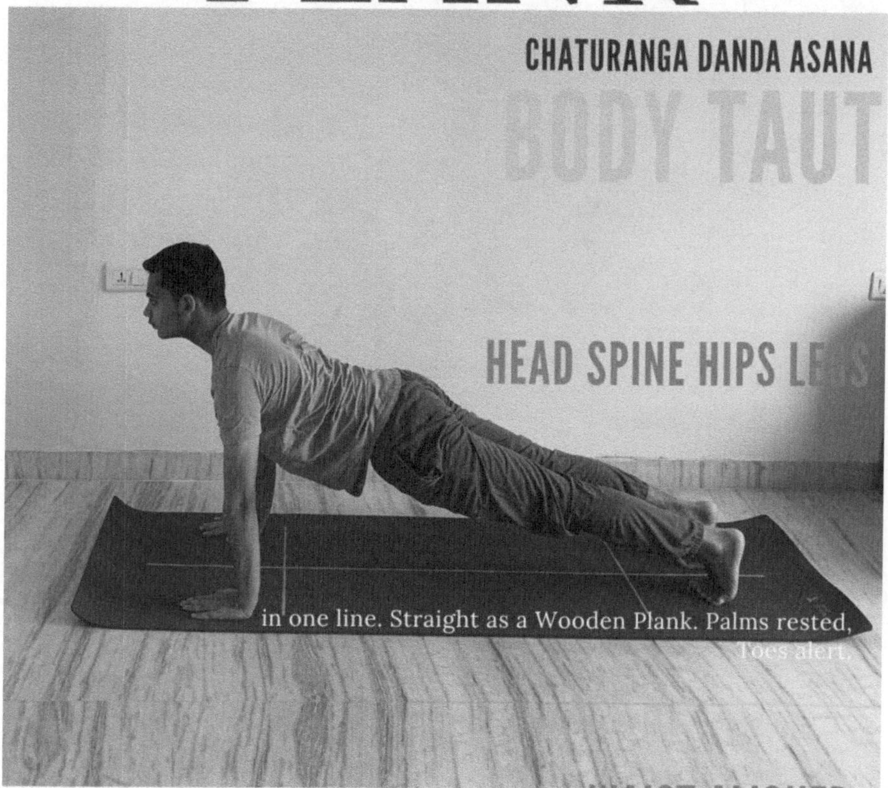
CHATURANGA DANDA ASANA
BODY TAUT
HEAD SPINE HIPS
in one line. Straight as a Wooden Plank. Palms rested,
Toes alert,

WAIST ALIGNED

Maintain focus on Straightness,
make each breath smooth
s l o w quiver-free

POSE FOR 2 BREATHS

06 Ashtanga Pranaam – Sashtanga Namaskar

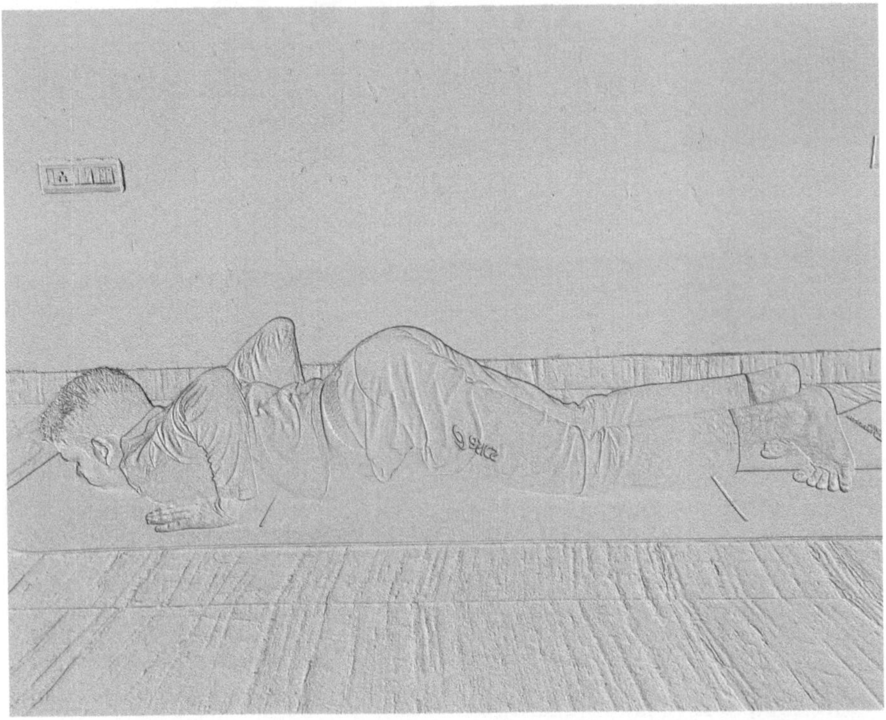

06 Ashtanga Pranaam

Without shifting the palms or feet from Pose 5

- Drop your Knees to the floor.
- Allow the Chest to rest on the ground
- Chin also rested on the ground
- Ensure that the Waist is in the Air
- One's linga is not touching the Earth during prostration.
- Observe the ambience and observe the silence.
- Allow the breath to become slow and deep.

PROSTRATE

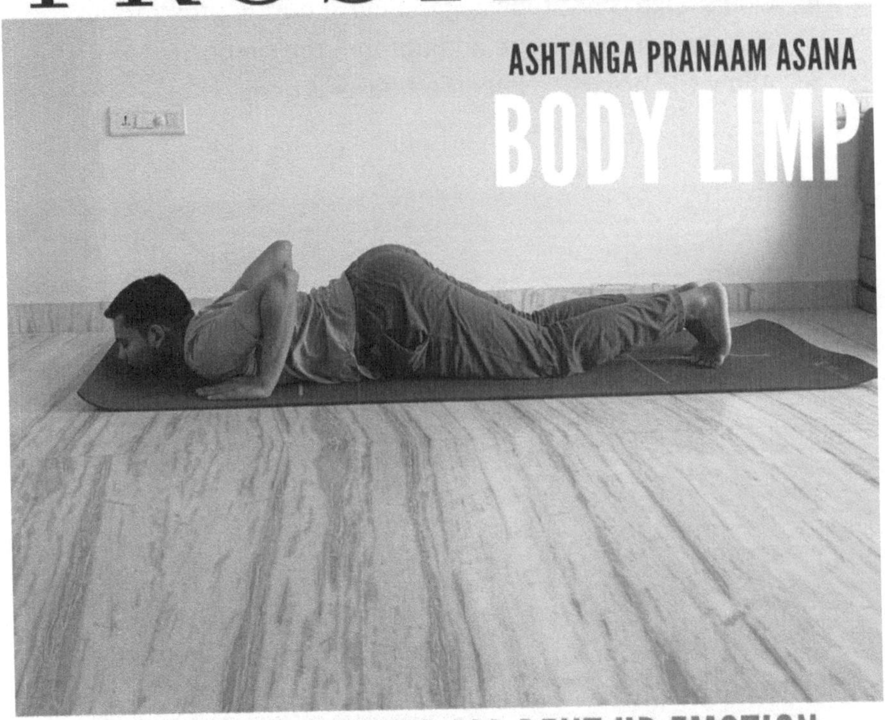

SURRENDER WASHES ALL PENT UP EMOTION
CLEANSES TO THE CORE

PROSTRATE

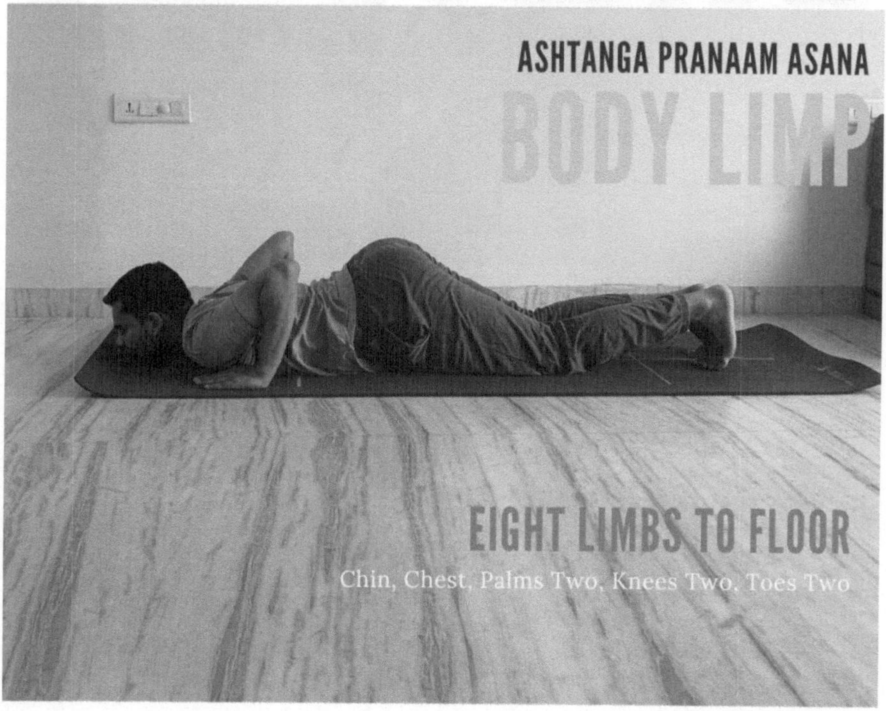
ASHTANGA PRANAAM ASANA
BODY LIMP
EIGHT LIMBS TO FLOOR
Chin, Chest, Palms Two, Knees Two, Toes Two

WAIST LIFTED

Maintain focus on uplifted waist, make each breath smooth s l o w quiver-free

POSE FOR 2 BREATHS

07 Cobra – Bhujang Asana

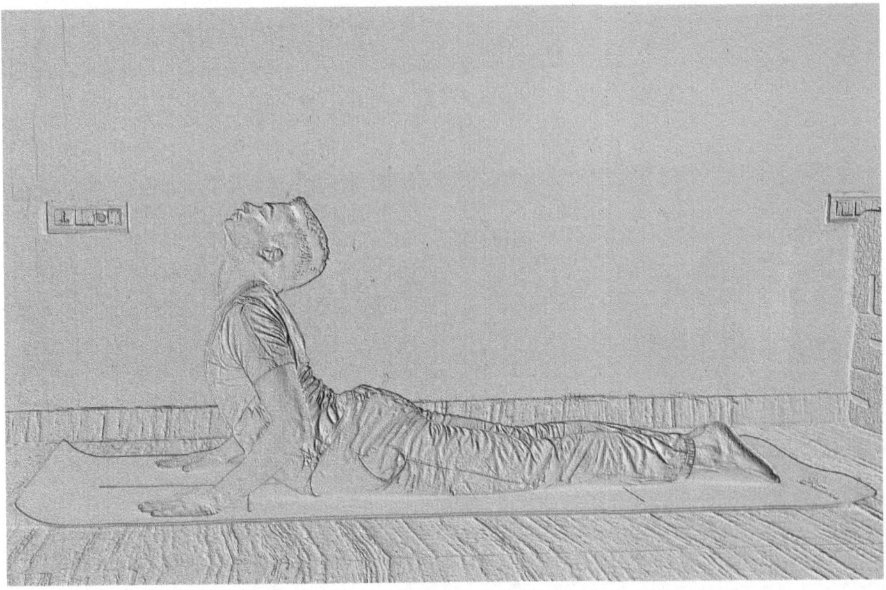

07 Cobra Pose

Without shifting the palms from Pose 6

- Drop your feet to rest on the floor.
- Allow the legs to rest on the ground
- Bring the Waist down to touch the ground
- With the weight on both palms, slowly lift the Chest
- Lift the torso only till the Nabhi Navel Center.
- Finally tilt the head back, look up towards the ceiling or. the mild Sun in the early morning dawn Sky.
- Observe the ambience and observe the silence.
- Allow the breath to become slow and deep.

COBRA

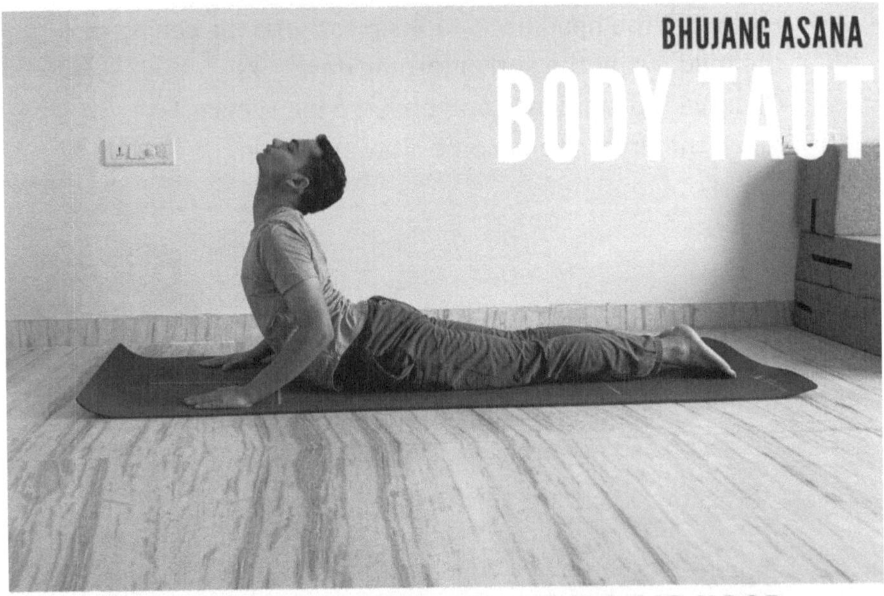

ALERT YET RELAXED AS A COBRA'S HOOD
KEEPS ALL WEAKNESS AT BAY

COBRA

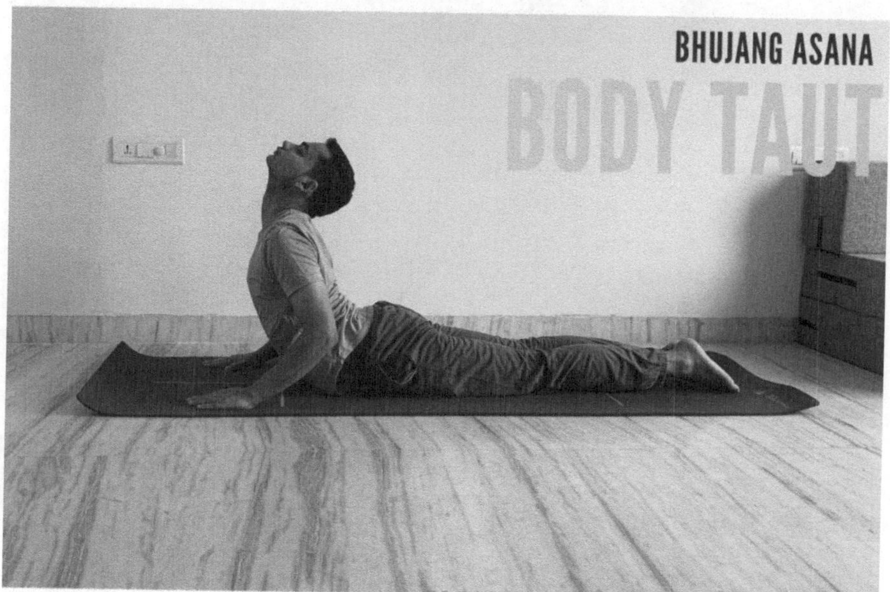

BHUJANG ASANA

BODY TAUT

NAVEL TO FEET ON FLOOR

Elbows Bent, Shoulders away from ears, Head tilted.

CHEST PROUD

Maintain focus on lumbar low back, make each breath smooth s l o w quiver-free

POSE FOR 2 BREATHS

08 Downward Dog – Adho Mukha Svan Asana

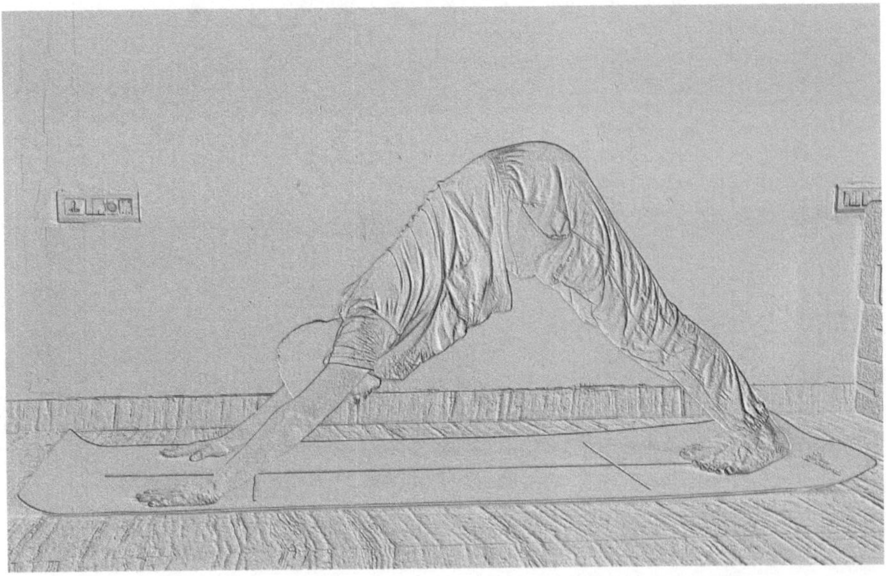

08 Downward Facing Dog Pose

Without shifting the palms from Pose 7

- Anchor the feet firmly and,
- Lift the torso all the way into an equilateral triangle.
- May readjust the distance between the palms and feet by walking the feet only, keeping the palms anchored.
- Allow the heels to rise just a bit
- The entire body is an inverted V shape
- Observe the ambience and observe the silence.
- Allow the breath to become slow and deep.

FACING DOG

DOWNWARD

BODY FIRM

ADHO MUKHA SVAN ASANA

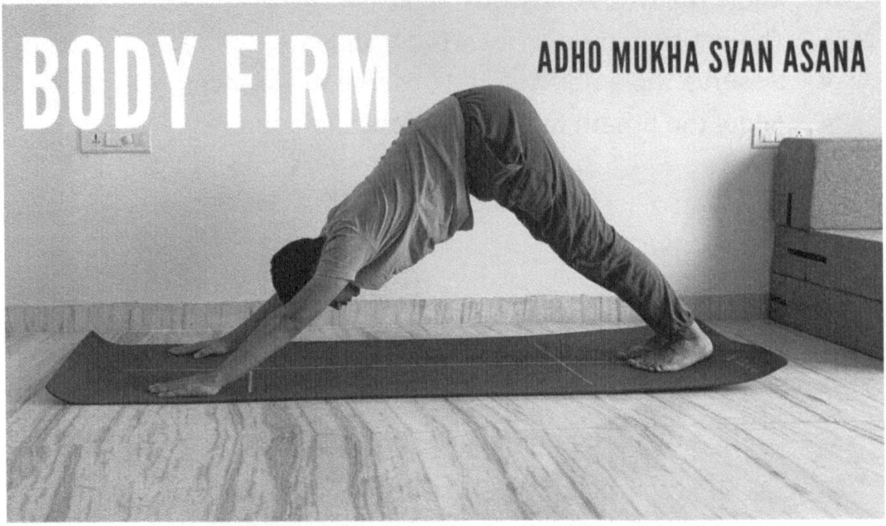

GEOMETRIC SHAPES ARE SACRED

MATH MAKES MY MIND SHARP

FACING DOG

DOWNWARD

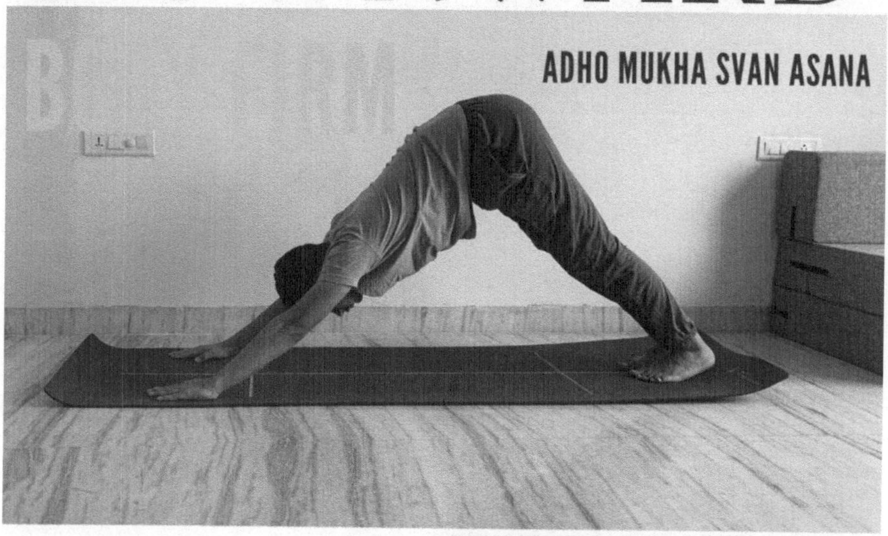

ADHO MUKHA SVAN ASANA

EQUILATERAL TRIANGLE

Palms anchored. Heels slightly lifted. Knees straight.
Inverted V.

GEOMETRY CALLING

Maintain focus on Nabhi Navel,
make each breath
smooth s l o w quiver-free

POSE FOR 2 BREATHS

09 Right Leg Front – Ashva Sanchalana Asana

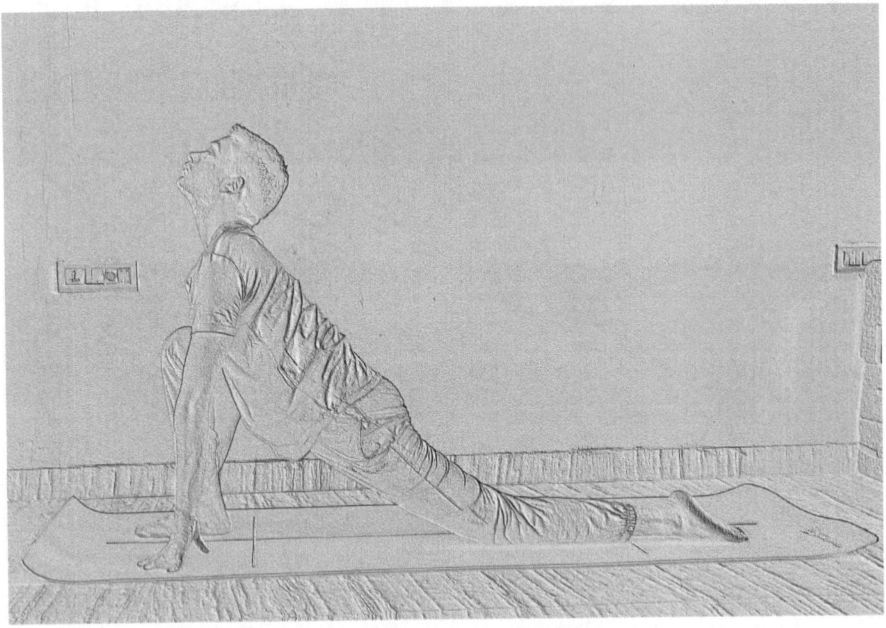

09 Horse Rider Pose – This is similar to pose 4 with change of leg

Without shifting the palms from Pose 8

- Bring the Right Leg forward and.
- Place the Right foot in between both palms
- Allow the left knee to touch the floor
- Allow the left foot to relax on the floor
- Now tilt the head back, look up to the ceiling or the mild Sun in the early morning dawn Sky.
- Observe the ambience and observe the silence.
- Allow the breath to become slow and deep.

FRONT

RIGHT LEG

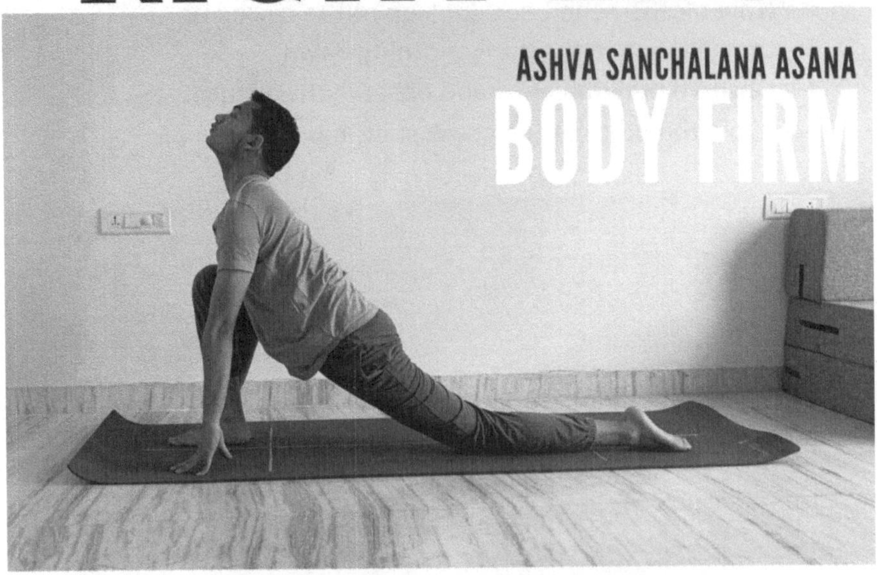

HORSEPOWER RATED FIGURE
SWIFTNESS GUARANTEED

FRONT

RIGHT LEG

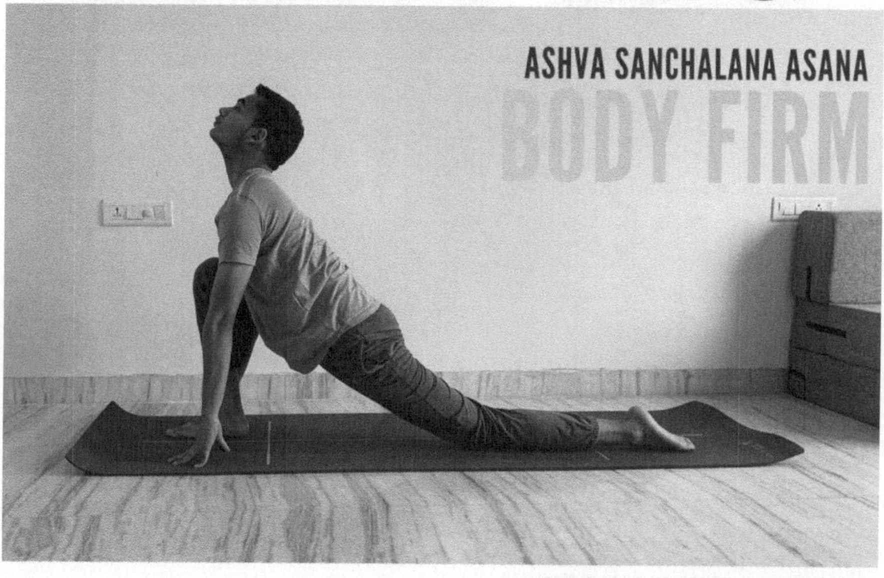

HORSE RIDER POSE

Right Foot anchored in between both Palms. Left foot relaxed, left knee on the floor.

FLEET FOOTED

Maintain focus on body balance, make each breath smooth s l o w quiver-free

POSE FOR 2 BREATHS

10 Left Leg Front – Hasta Pada Asana

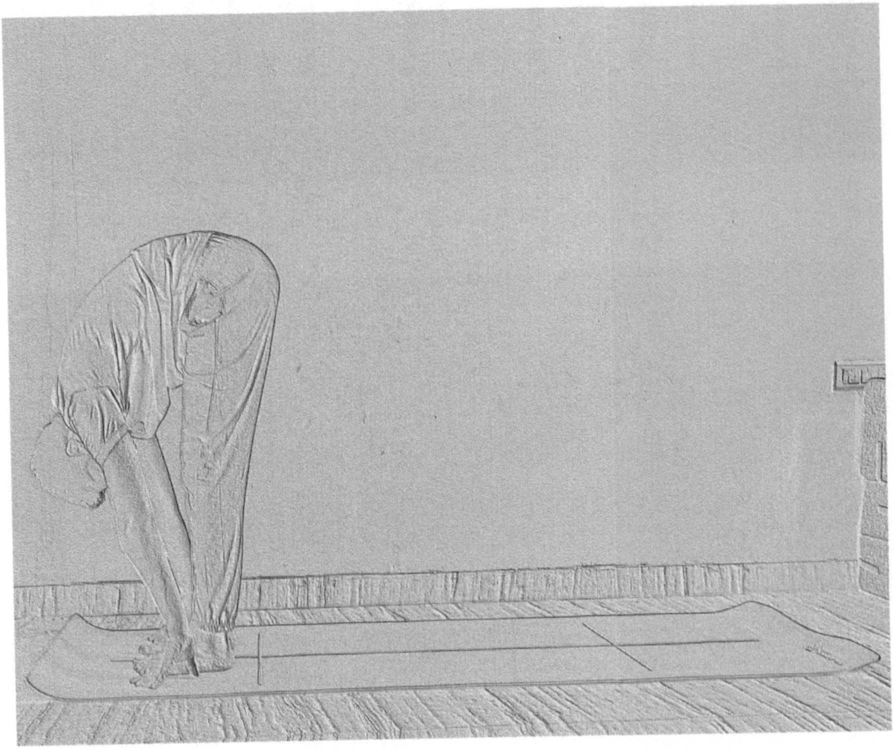

10 Standing Forward Bend – This is identical to Pose 3

Without shifting the palms from Pose 9

- Bring the Left Leg forward and.
- Place the left foot in between both palms next to the Right foot
- Maintain a gap of 5-6 inches between both feet
- Keeping the palms touching the floor,
- Rise up and make the Knees straight, flexing the leg muscles
- Allow the head to come close to the knees
- Maintain contact of the palms with the ground.
- Observe the ambience and observe the silence.
- Allow the breath to become slow and deep.

STANDING BEND

FORWARD

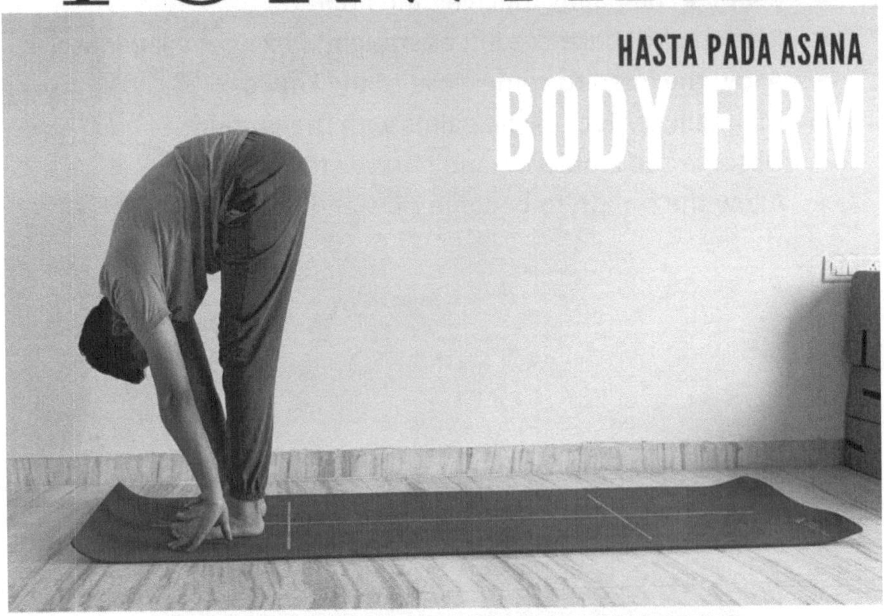

KNEES CHARGED I GROW BY LEAPS & BOUNDS, FULFILLING ALL AIMS

STANDING

BEND

FORWARD

HASTA PADA ASANA

BODY FIRM

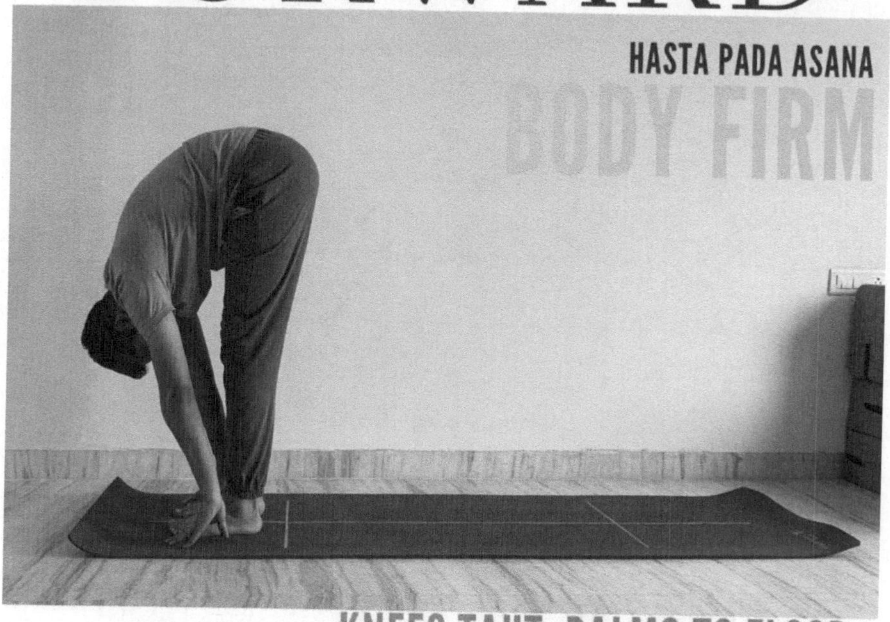

KNEES TAUT, PALMS TO FLOOR

Head bowed, Feet steady, Knee muscles in play

WAIST BEND

Maintain focus on knees,
make each breath
smooth s l o w quiver-free

POSE FOR 2 BREATHS

11 Up and Back – Hasta Uttana Asana

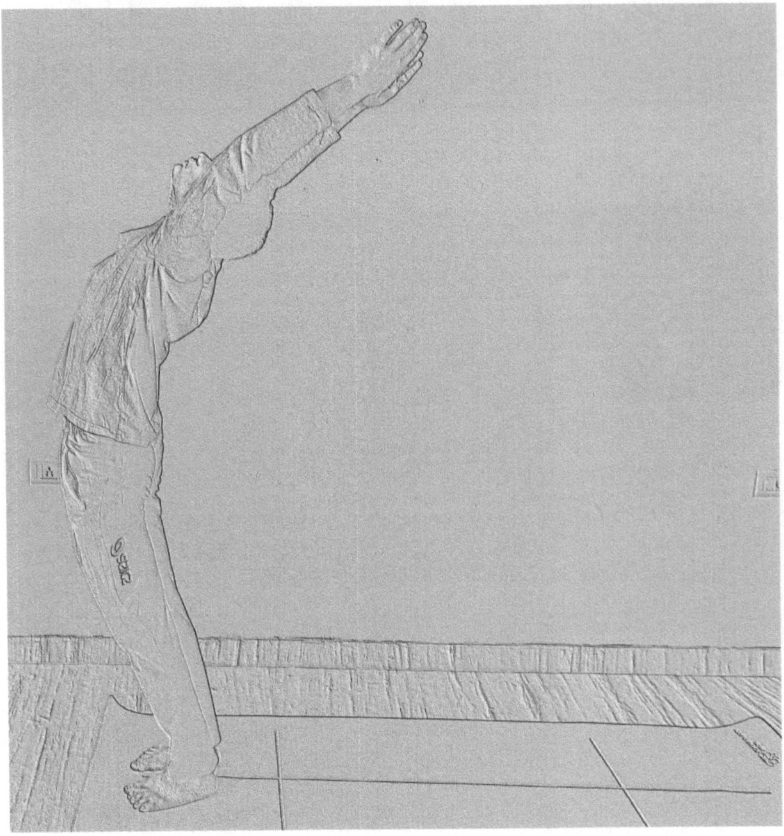

11 Raised Arms Up and Back – This is identical to Pose 2

Without shifting the feet from Pose 10

- Slowly rise UP from the Waist
- Keep the head in between the arms,
- Maintain both arms parallel to each other
- Straighten all the way Up to standing position
- Then continue moving from the Waist
- Bend back a bit from the Waist
- Allow the torso to be in a nice arch
- Look up to the ceiling or
  the mild Sun in the early morning dawn Sky.
- Observe the ambience and observe the silence.
- Allow the breath to become slow and deep.

ARMS RAISED

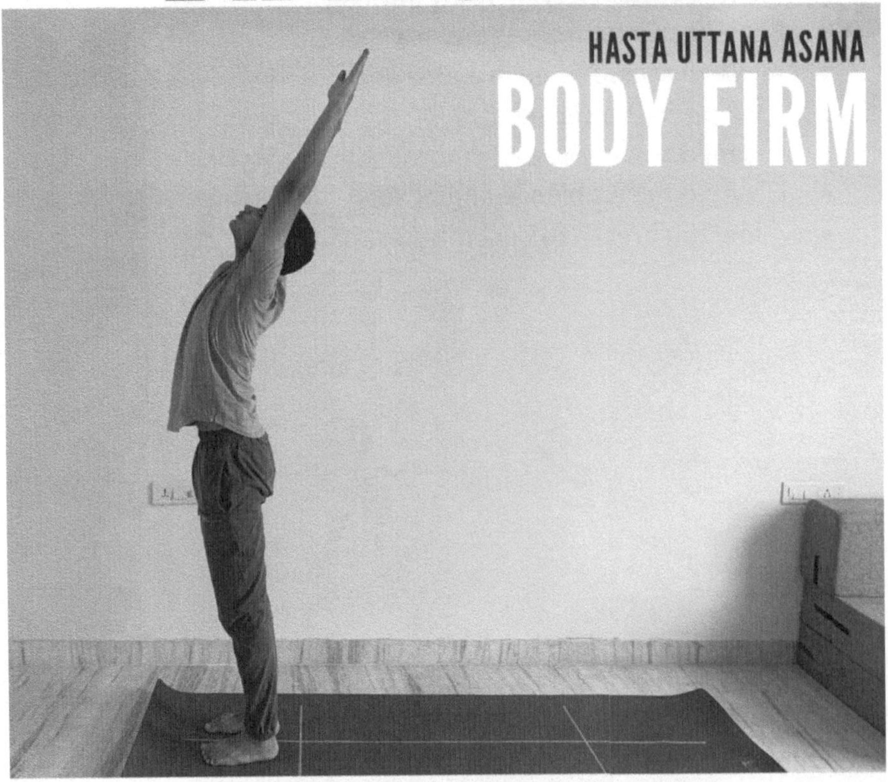

UP ABOVE THE WORLD SO HIGH
LIKE A DIAMOND IN THE SKY

ARMS

RAISED

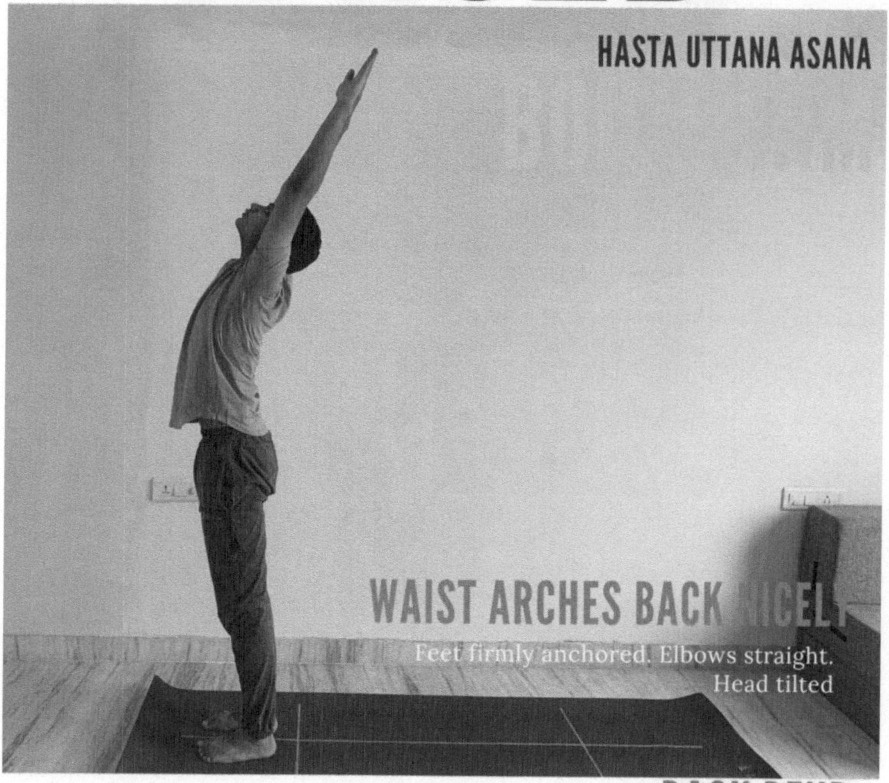
HASTA UTTANA ASANA
WAIST ARCHES BACK
Feet firmly anchored. Elbows straight.
Head tilted

BACK BEND

Maintain focus on Nabhi Navel,
make each breath
smooth s l o w quiver-free

POSE FOR 2 BREATHS

12 Namaste – Pranaam Asana

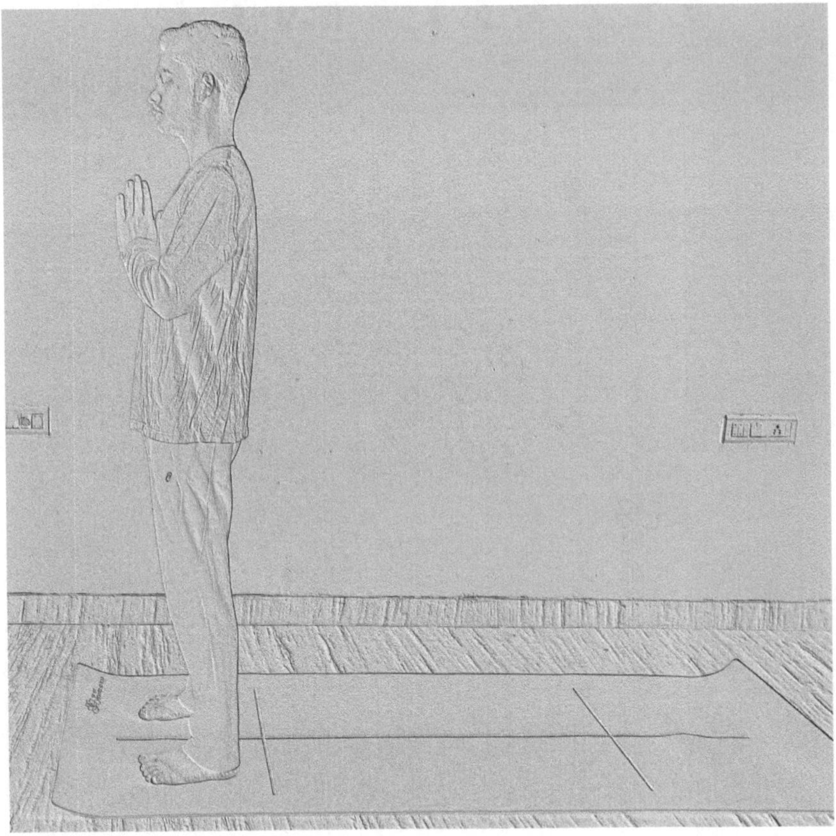

12 Namaste – This is identical to Pose 1

Without shifting the feet from Pose 11

- Slowly bring the arms down from the sides
- To chest level and join both palms
- Take a moment to go within.
- Observe the ambience and observe the silence.
- Allow the breath to become slow and deep
- May bend forward just a bit in reverence. Or simply feel it in the heart.

NAMASTE

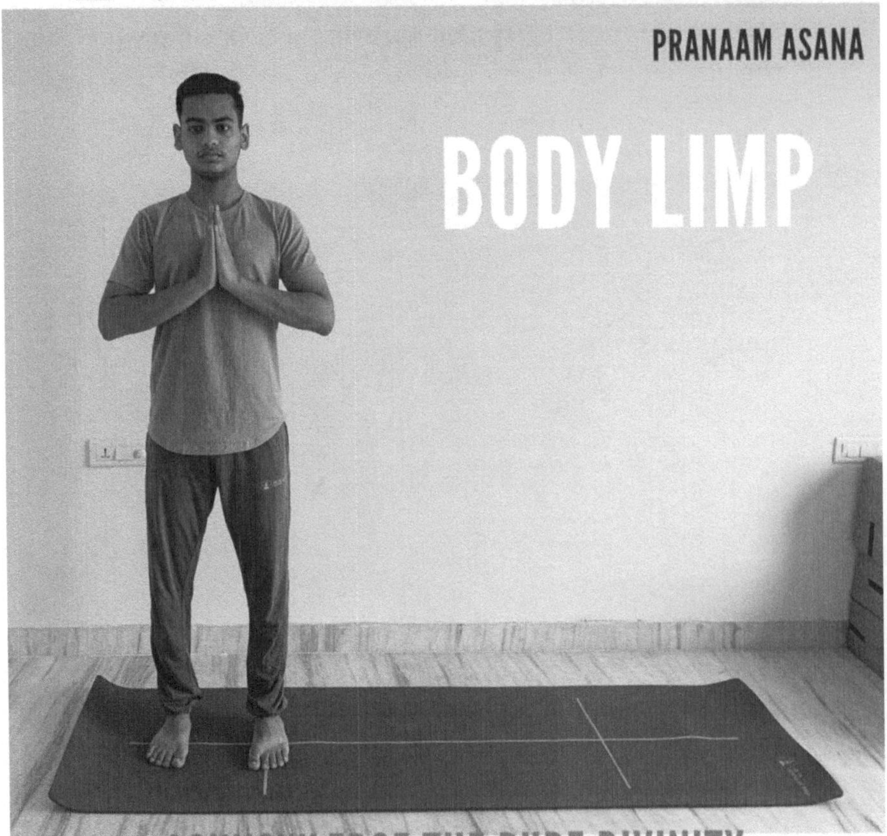

ACKNOWLEDGE THE PURE DIVINITY
OUTSIDE & INSIDE

NAMASTE

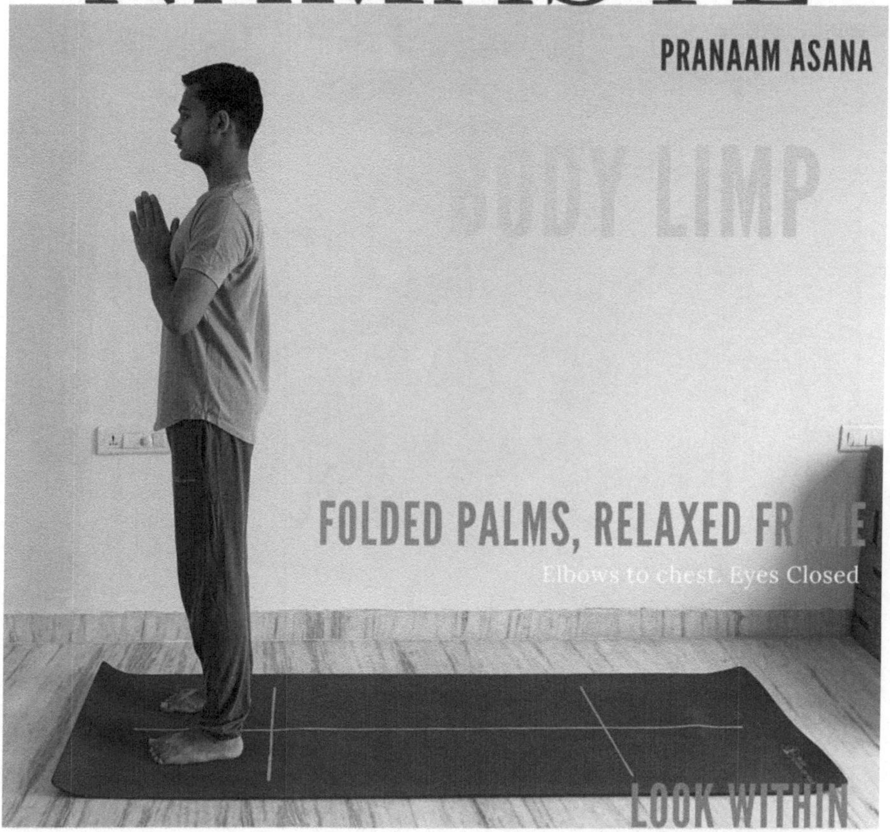
PRANAAM ASANA
BODY LIMP
FOLDED PALMS, RELAXED FR
Elbows to chest. Eyes Closed
LOOK WITHIN

Maintain focus on Gratefulness,
make each breath smooth
s l o w quiver-free

POSE FOR 2 BREATHS

Sculpted in Bronze

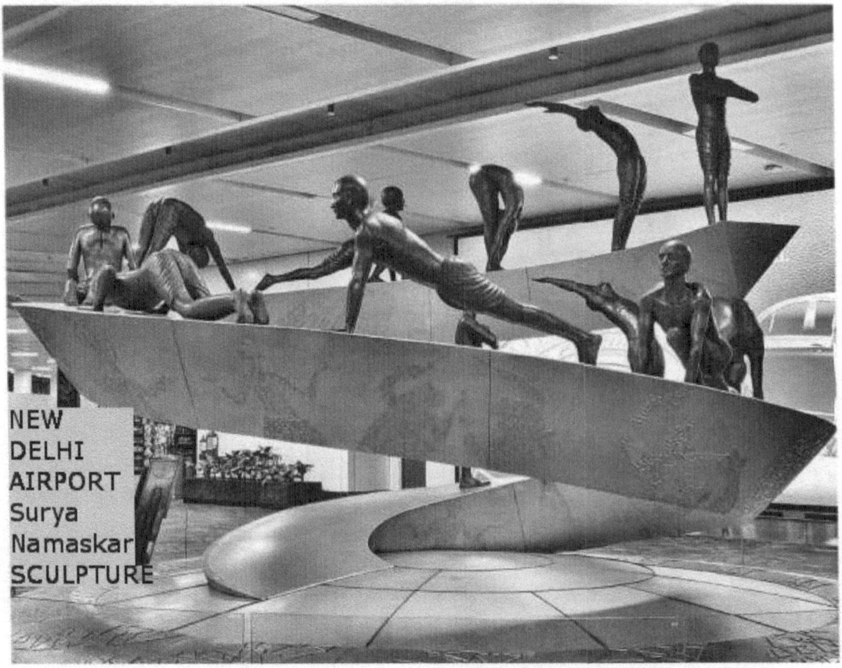

PRONE

VISHNU

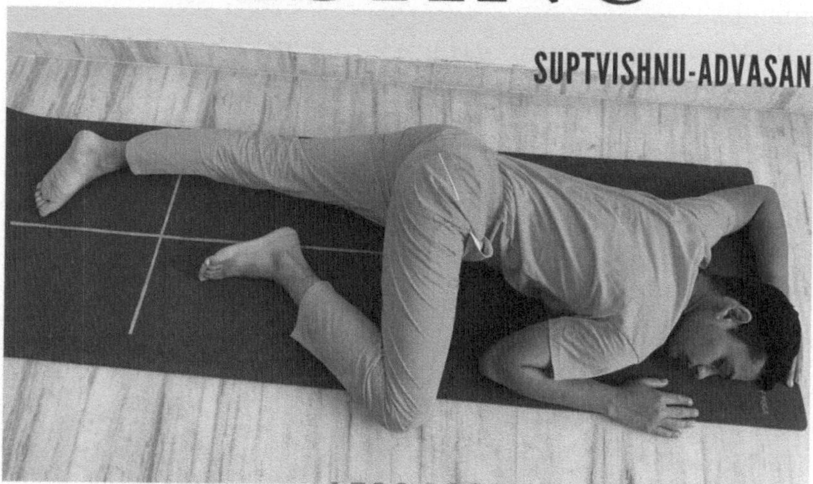

SUPTVISHNU-ADVASANA

BODY LIMP

LEGS LOOSE ONE KNEE BENT

Neck loose. Face Relaxed.
Delicate sleep

PALMS OPEN TO FLOOR

Let go the focus, make each breath smooth s l o w quiver-free

POSE AS LONG AS COMFORTABLE

Yoga Nidra

We look for so much attention outside. We go crazy trying to please someone. In our Yogic tradition there is a brilliant method of taking a conscious shower that harmonizes each body part and actually raises our charm to a degree that cosmetics and body sprays can never do.

Remember –

- the key to efficient performance at the workplace
- the magic in engaging relationships

is deep and sufficient relaxation.

Yog Nidra Sadhguru Guided Meditation For Sleep
https://www.youtube.com/watch?v=veeAGGq577s

Yoga Nidra - Guided Meditation for Sleep & Relaxation – Sri Sri
https://www.youtube.com/watch?v=zLJu3wQA1Ko

Yoga Nidra - Swami Niranjanananda Saraswati
https://www.youtube.com/watch?v=04qZCaKFSWc

Meditation

It goes without saying that Meditation twice a day for a few minutes shall integrate and bind all our activities, enhance our immunity greatly, and lead to long term material success that is stable.

Meditation is simply honoring the unknown. Getting in touch with the cosmos, the infinite vastness that fulfills all and showers pleasurable bliss.

Memory and Meditation –
A Neuroscientist in Conversation with Sri Sri
https://www.youtube.com/watch?v=h7lPFXJCvKI

Meditate with Gurudev
https://www.srisriravishankar.org/live/
https://www.youtube.com/playlist?list=PLH-0HZ0SQ_PEYRcjsRvxivVhGPk2iT6iZ

10 minute Guided Meditation for Beginners
https://www.youtube.com/watch?v=TWbiDzi-rQc

Glow of the Candle
https://www.youtube.com/watch?v=-vrcUArnd-w

Meditate with your Breath
https://www.youtube.com/watch?v=SShjEQfK-w0

Healing Flute Music
https://www.youtube.com/watch?v=unuiaZleQ5c

Technology of Spirituality – A talk by Khurshed Batliwala
https://www.youtube.com/watch?v=I9aR_xfm-gE

Sequence

Stand Tall 0

Do a bit of standing jog and move all your body parts and joints. Flex and loosen your shoulder and neck muscles. Rotate your waist, ankles, toes.

Then stand limp with arms hanging loosely by the sides.
Feet apart, well anchored.

Tadasana. Steady Tall Pose. Mountain Pose.

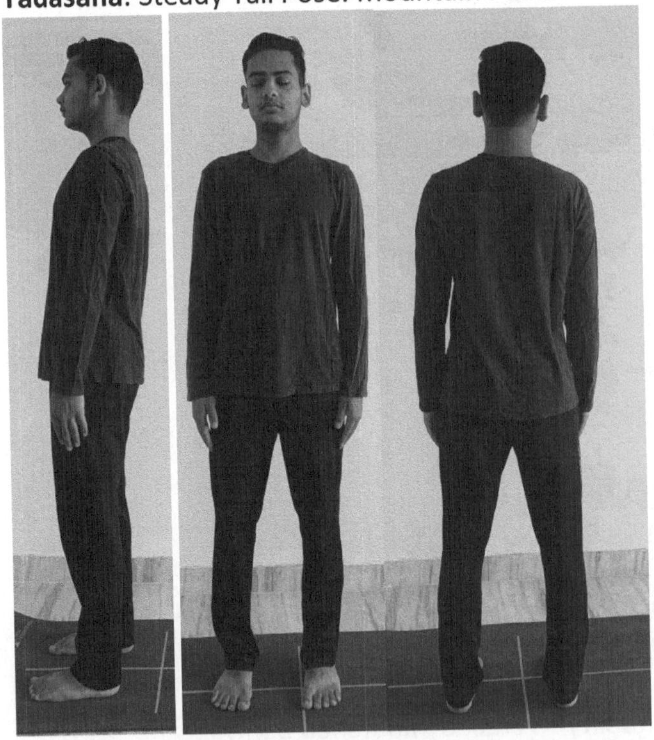

MOUNTAIN

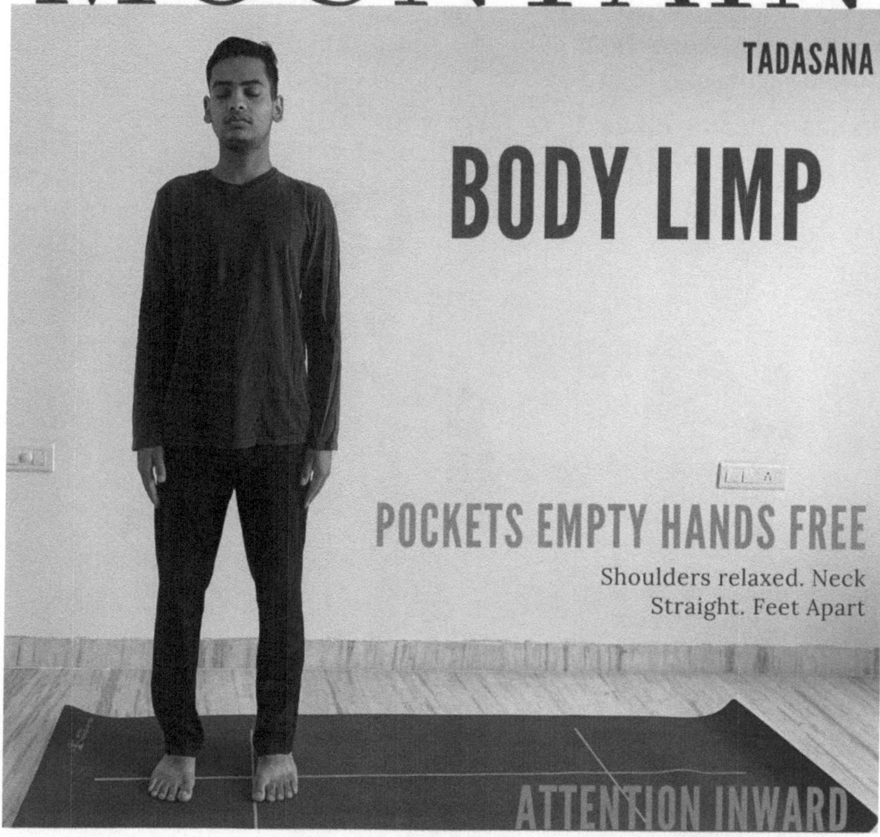

Maintain focus on Body Tension, make each breath smooth s l o w quiver-free

POSE AS LONG AS COMFORTABLE

1 Breathe IN Namaste

Feet apart, body limp, easy in the mind.

Hands come up and palms join. Honor yourself, Honor the ambience.

Smile and gently close the Eyes.
Take a couple of Deep Breaths.

Breathe IN Breathe OUT.

Pranaam Asana. Prayer Pose.

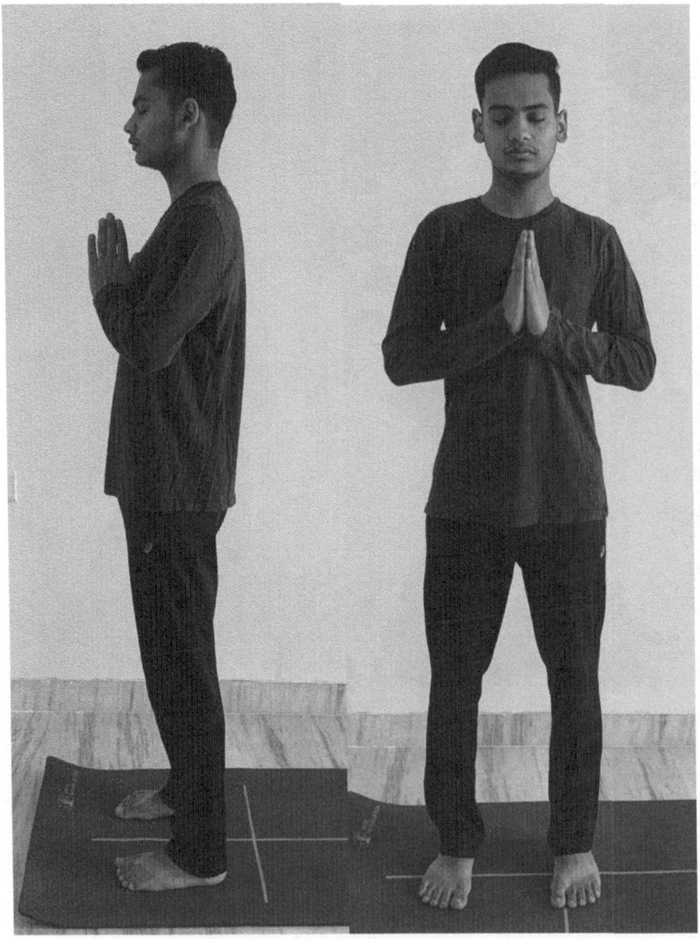

2 Breathe IN, Up and Back

Breathe IN. Hands separate, arms open

Go UP and Back. A Gentle arch.

Neck, Head aligned in between the arms.

Take couple of Deep Breaths.

Hasta Uttana Asana. Raised Arms Pose

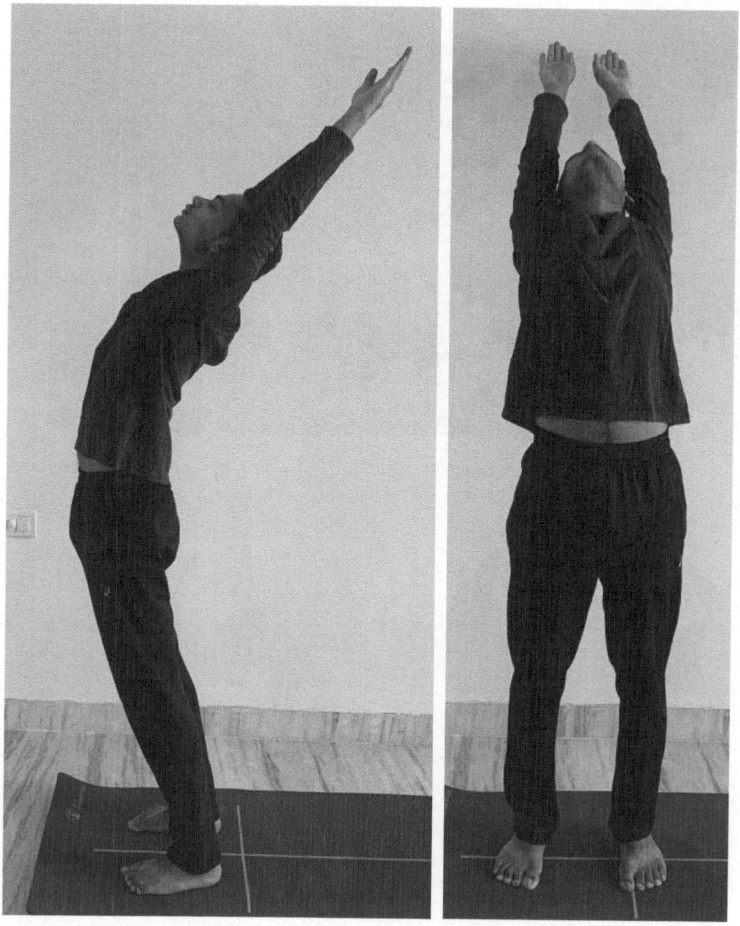

3 Breathe OUT, Forward and Down

Breathe OUT. Bend Forward and Down. From the waist.

Keep Neck, Head, Arms aligned while going down.

Touch the floor, Knees are Straight.
Take couple of Deep Breaths.

Hasta Pada Asana. Hands to Feet Pose.

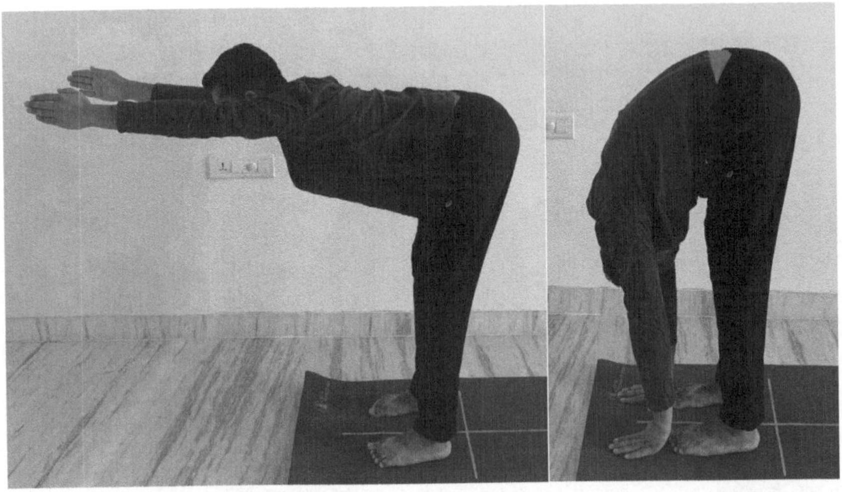

4 Breathe IN, Right Leg Back

Position the palms besides the feet on either side.

Breathe IN. Right Leg goes Back. Right Knee touches the floor. Tilt the Neck, Look UP, a Gentle Arch.

Take couple of Deep Breaths.

Ashva Sanchalana Asana. Horse Rider Equestrian Pose.

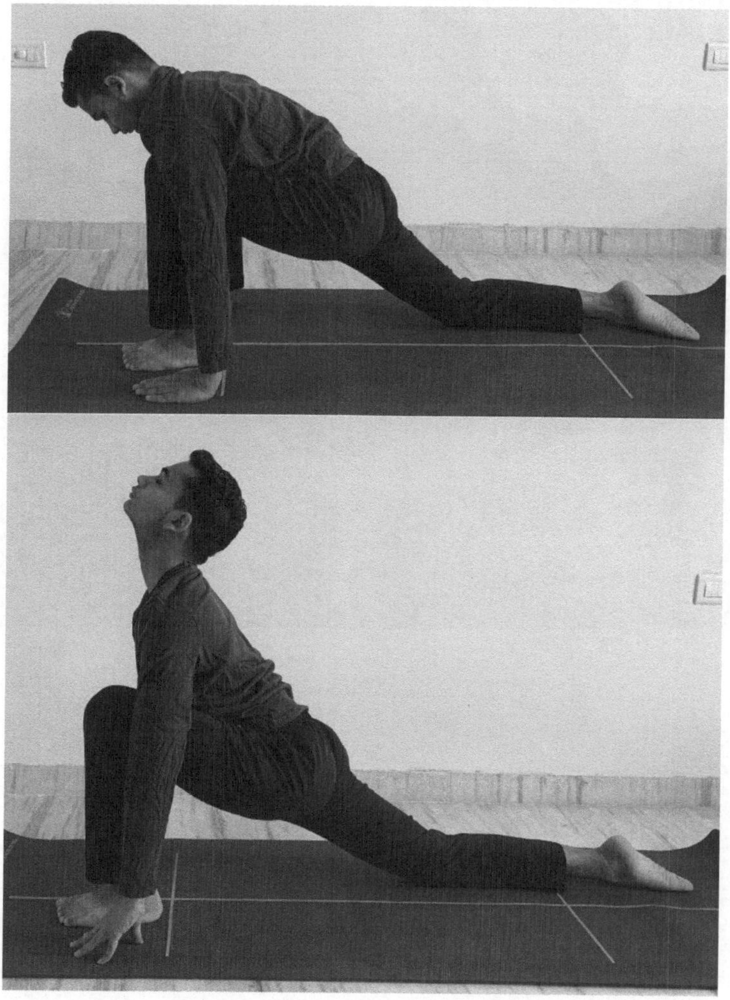

5 Breathe IN, Other Leg Back

Breathe IN. Other Leg goes Back. Knees off the floor.
Entire body in one line.

Neck and Head and Waist in one slanting line.
Anchored on palms and toes, the Four limbs.

Take couple of Deep Breaths.

Chaturanga Danda Asana. Plank Pose.

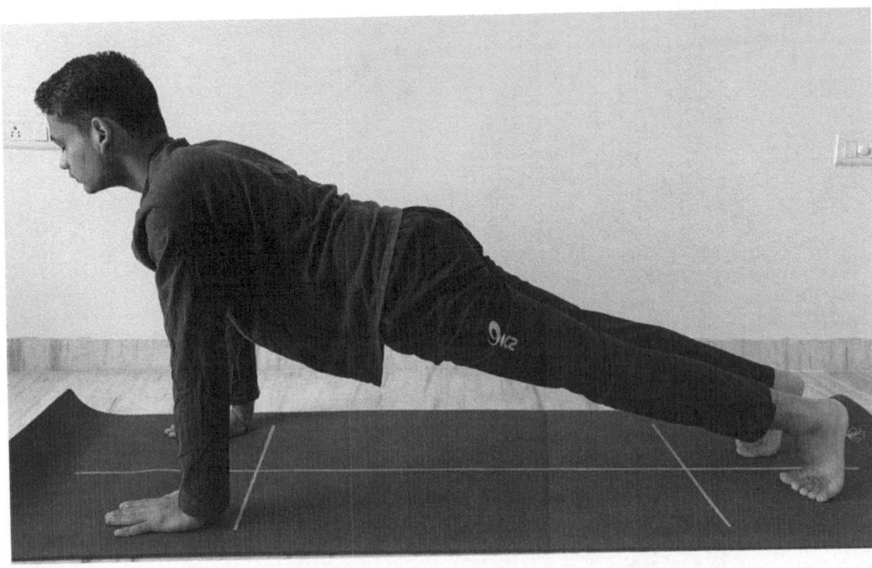

6 Breathe OUT, Body to Ground

Breathe OUT. Knees drop to the floor.
Body arches back and rears forward to rest Chin on the floor.

Arms close to the body, palms near the shoulders.
Waist off the ground, our linga is in the air.

Eight points of contact – 2 feet, 2 knees, 2 palms, chest and chin.

Take couple of Deep Breaths.

Sashtanga Namaskar. **Ashtanga Pranaam**. Prostration Pose.

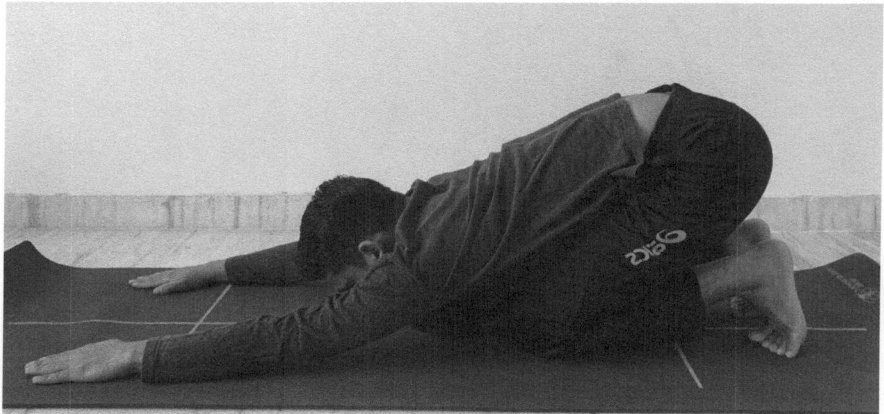

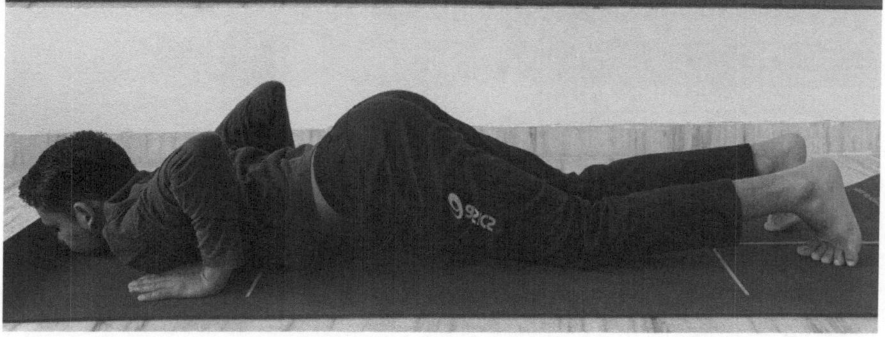

7 Breathe IN, Lift Up to Cobra

Breathe IN. Chest rises up slowly. Head Tilts back. Look Skywards. Body arches nicely to flex all the back muscles and align the spine.

Arms close to the body, palms near the shoulders.
Lift only till the Nabhi, Navel center.

Waist, Legs, Knees, Feet on the floor.

Take couple of Deep Breaths.

Bhujang Asana. Cobra Pose.

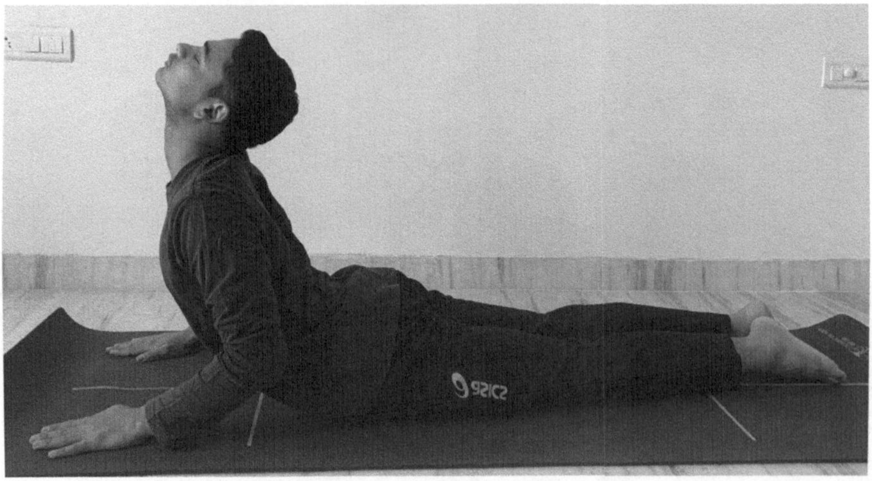

8 Breathe IN to Downward Dog

Breathe OUT, chest comes down.
Breathe IN, torso raises Up in equilateral triangle shape.

Palms and feet firmly anchored. Heels may be slightly off.

Take couple of Deep Breaths.

Adho Mukha Svan Asana. Downward Facing Dog Pose.

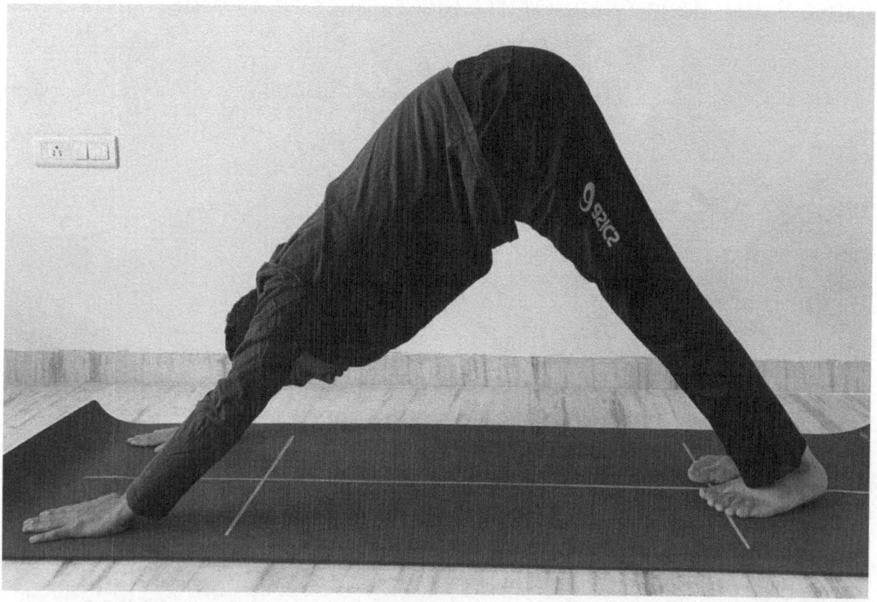

9 Breathe IN, Right Leg Front

Breathe IN, Right Leg comes to front in between the palms. Head Tilts Up, look Skywards. Body is in a gentle arch.

Left Foot resting on the floor. Left Knee touching the ground.

This Pose is similar to Pose 4, with change in leg.
Take couple of Deep Breaths.

Ashva Sanchalana Asana. Horse Rider Equestrian Pose.

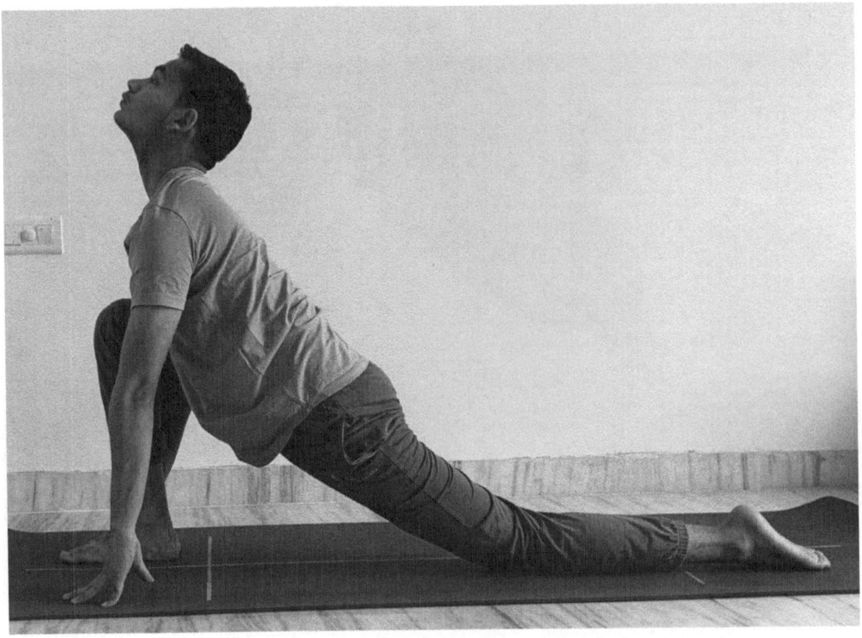

10 Breathe IN, Other Leg Front

Breathe IN, Left Leg comes to front in between the palms.
Knees become straight, Forward Bend.

Head comes close to knees, palms on the ground.

This Pose is identical to Pose 3.
Take couple of Deep Breaths.

Hasta Pada Asana. Hands to Feet Pose.

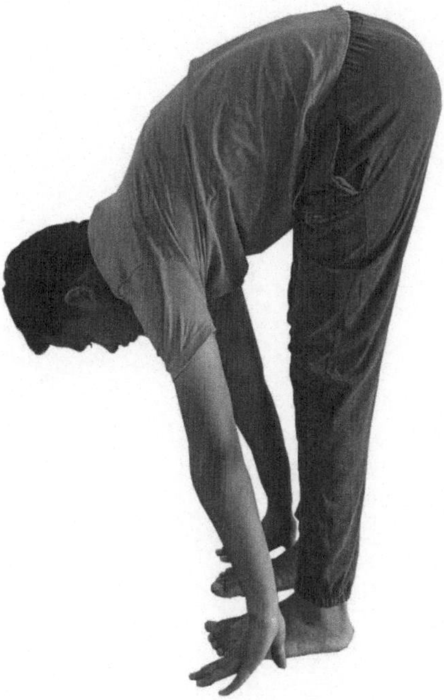

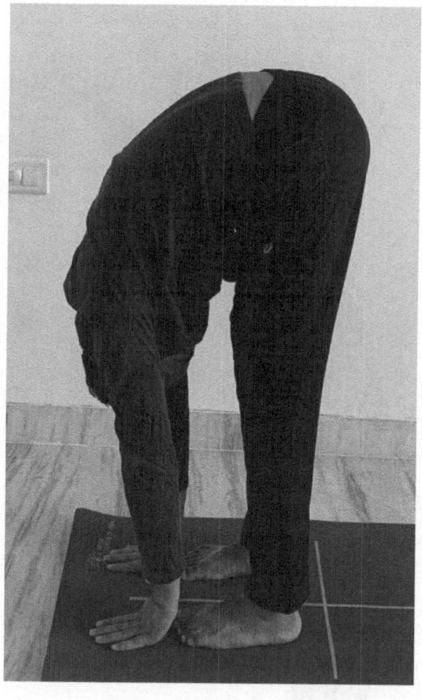

11 Breathe IN go Up and Back

Breathe IN, go Up and Back.
Rise from the Waist, keeping head aligned in between the arms.

Neck and Head firm. Waist goes back. Torso is in a beautiful arch.

This Pose is identical to Pose 2.
Take couple of Deep Breaths.

Hasta Uttana Asana. Raised Arms Pose.

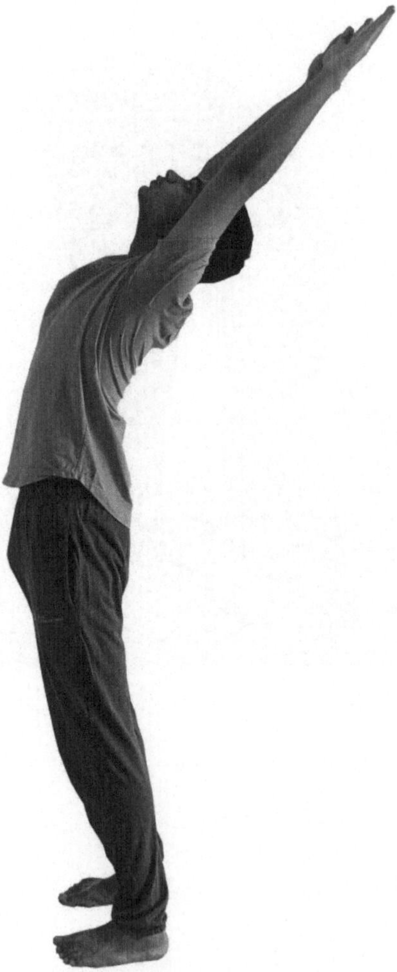

12 Breathe OUT Namaste

Breathe OUT, arms come down from the sides.
Palms join, body straight and limp.

Go Inwards. Become Grateful. Honor the creation. Honor thyself.

This Pose is identical to Pose 1.
Take couple of Deep Breaths.

Pranaam Asana. Prayer Pose.

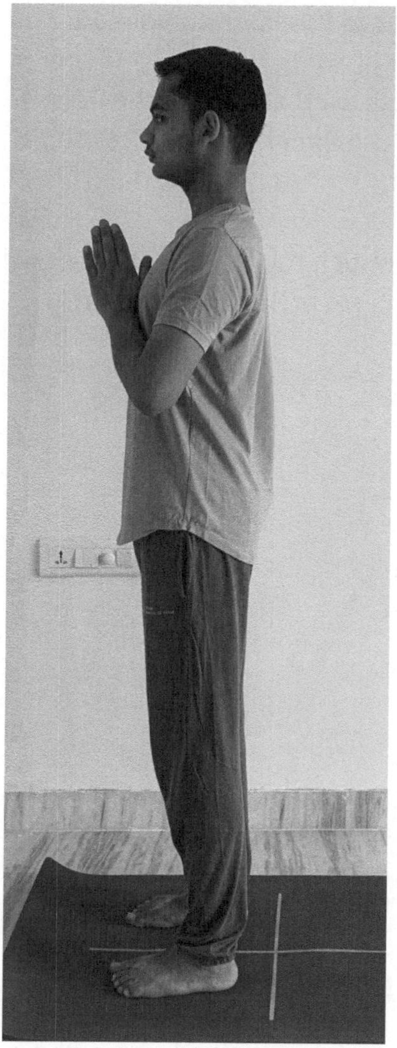

Let Go 13

Breathe IN, hands come down and hang loosely by the sides.

Be with yourself. Be with your own experience.

This Pose is identical to Pose 0. Take couple of Deep Breaths.

Tadasana. Standing Tall Pose.

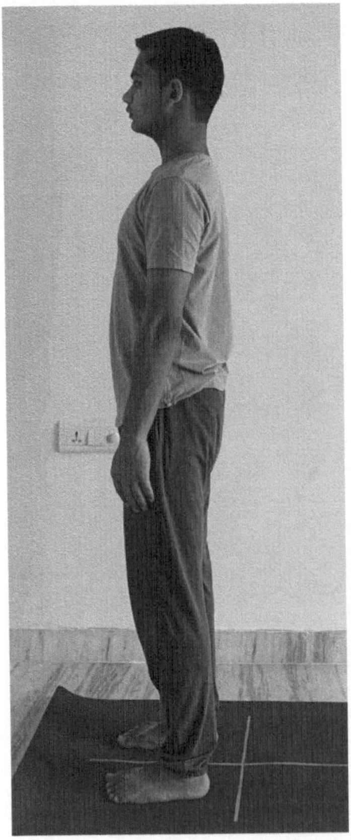

When we do multiple rounds of Surya Namaskar, then we skip this step and go straight to Pose 2 from pose 12.

In that case we then repeat the Pose 4 with Left Leg Back, and Pose 9 with Left Leg Front.

Doing two such rounds of 12 poses each makes one set of Surya Namaskar.

After Ending

May lie down in Shavasana

Eyes closed.
Loosen and adjust all joints and muscles. Then become still. Make the breath soft.

Rest as long as needed. Then roll to the right side and sit up.

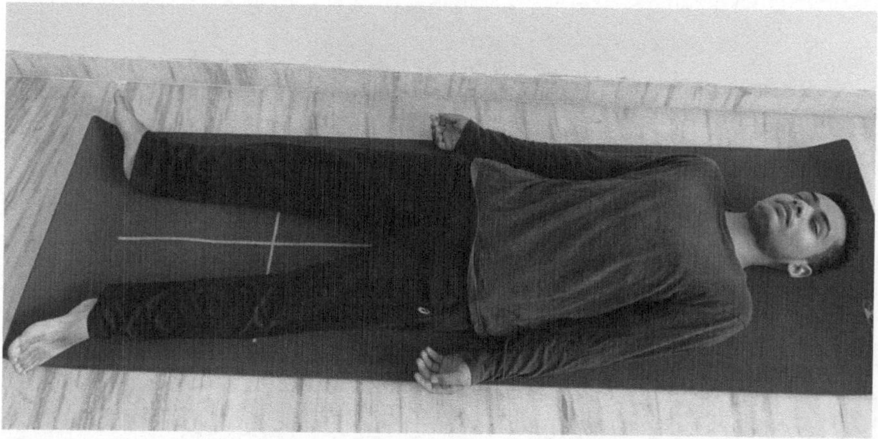

Grace is in Gratefulness

Smile freely. Offer your practice to the Great Lord. To your near and dear ones. And become Free.

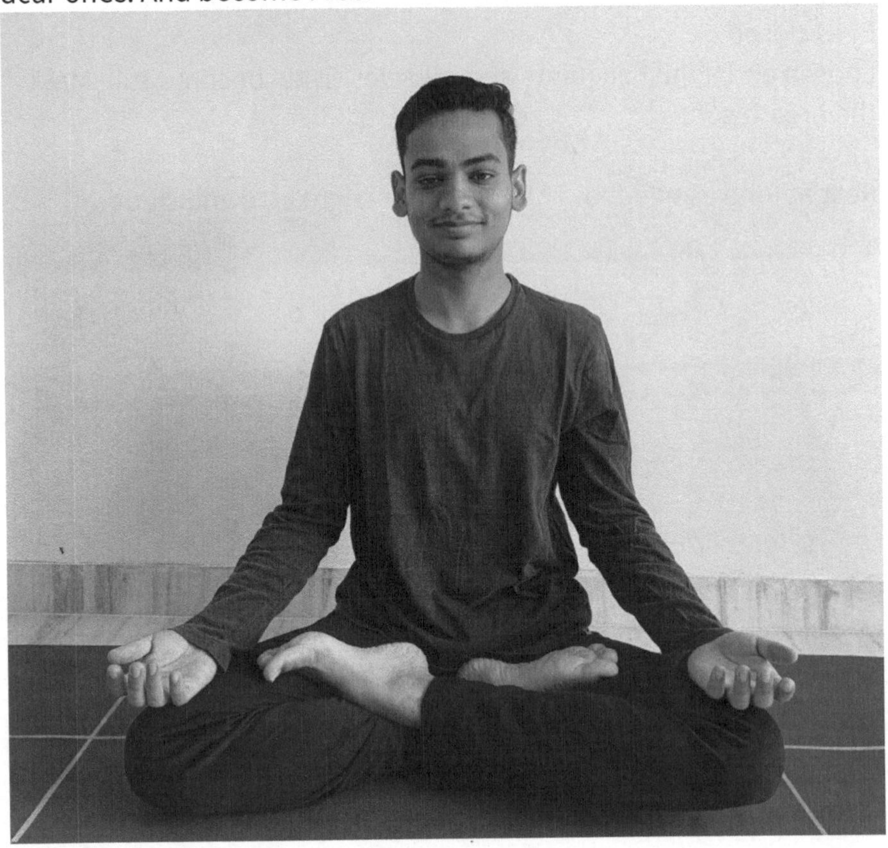

Roll up the Yogamat

For another day.

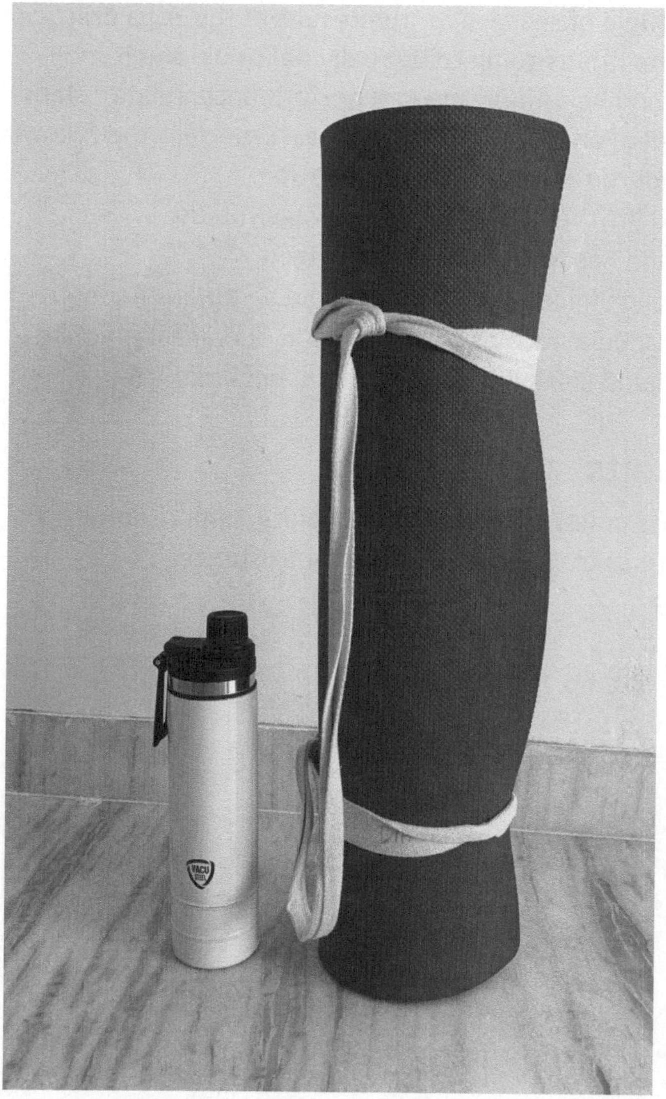

Significant Aspects

One notices something happening only after a few days. In fact the real smoothness in life takes a while to show up. It may take for e.g. 108 days or a couple of seasons for the results of the Yoga practice to bear fruit. But the fruit is going to be really delicious, and it shall reflect strongly and beautifully in work performance, relationships and general level of energy and cheerfulness. Especially the following aspects shall undergo a positive transformation.

- Flow and Rhythm in any creative things you do
- Timing and Rest gets properly managed
- Silence and Stillness writ conflicts and agitations happens
- Posture and Balance of both body and personality radiates
- Strength and Flexibility of both mind and body is felt

Regular Habits

Apart from asana practice, the following habits support our Yoga aura and nurture us from a deeper plane of existence.

- Chanting
- Prayer
- Lighting a Lamp
- Puja Havan Satsang Aarti

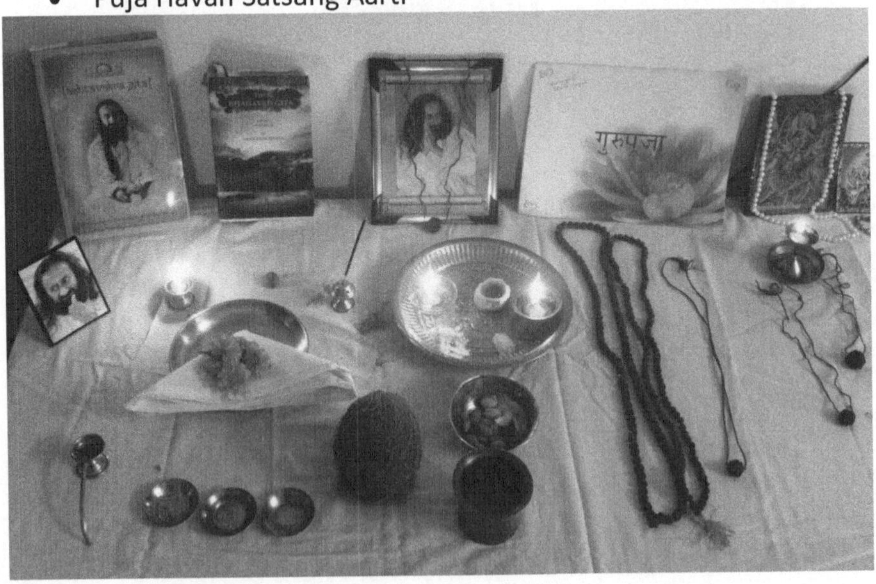

Guruji answers - Why is Puja Necessary?
https://www.youtube.com/watch?v=PuFqCrl8SX0

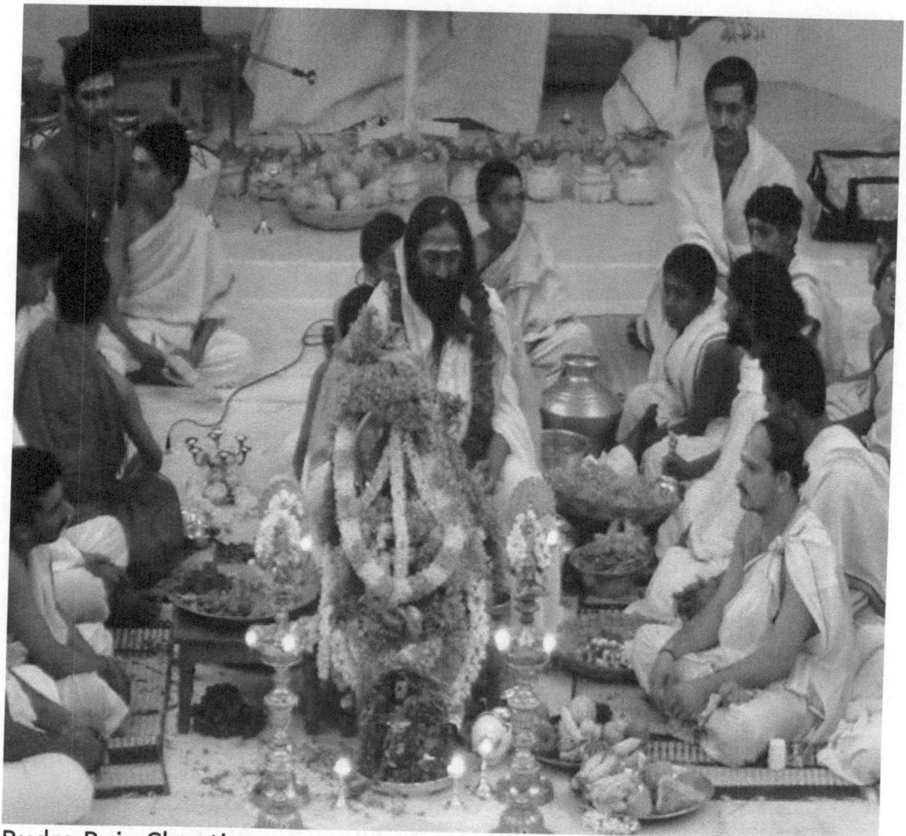

Rudra Puja Chanting
https://www.youtube.com/watch?v=QjsO4UVwsow

GuruPuja by Bhanu Didi
https://www.youtube.com/watch?v=htXI6Fommfw

Daily Watch

Food is a potential parameter that can make or break any target. For some reason, the scientific reasons behind eating a proper vegetarian diet has been long forgotten or overlooked. However it is slowly surfacing and being talked about in the medical circles and journals. Famous personalities are boldly implementing it, and their success is enough testimony for the same.

Ayurveda & Diet

Ayurveda is a safe mechanism to mix and match our diet as per our native constitution. It will prevent many ills and mood swings. It makes sense to get a pulse diagnosis nadi pariksha done. And it goes without saying that locally grown fresh fruits and vegetables, and A2 cow milk products should be a diet priority. Replacing white sugar with honey, jaggery, etc., sea salt with rock salt, and refined oils with cold pressed mustard or groundnut oil, such culinary methods make a remarkable turnaround in overall health levels.
https://www.artofliving.org/ayurveda

Vitamins

Due to the increased usage of mechanized farming, packaged foods, and high dosage of chemicals, colors, preservatives, or flavors in our eatables, the real essence of food is pushed far into the background. It just remains a belly fill without nourishment. So we must supplement our diet with Shakti Drops and other Ayurvedic concoctions.

Gurudev on Turmeric and Ginger and Giloye (Amruth balli)
https://www.youtube.com/watch?v=sYoCdmjkGlg

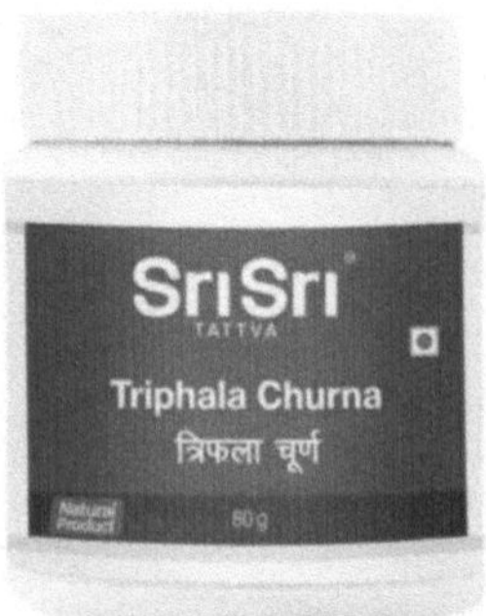

Eat a teaspoon of Triphala Churna with warm water at bedtime for a fortnight.

Wash your eyes daily with Triphala water for ten days.

Eye Care & Tooth Care

Eyes are ost beautiful and need to be kept functional till a ripe old age. We can wash them with triphala water that has been strained using a fine cloth. Simply add a teaspoon of triphala powder to a cup of plain water and leave overnight in a copper vessel.

Also, keep a tissue paper dipped in cool Rose water over the eyes and relax for a few minutes with eyes closed.

Sri Sri Shakti Drops
It is advisable to add 4 drops to a cup of water and drink regularly.
https://www.amazon.in/Sri-Ayurveda-Shakti-Drops-10/dp/B017IJGG44

Patanjali Dant Kanti Manjan
https://www.patanjaliayurved.net/product/natural-personal-care/dental-care/advanced-dant-kanti-manjan/870

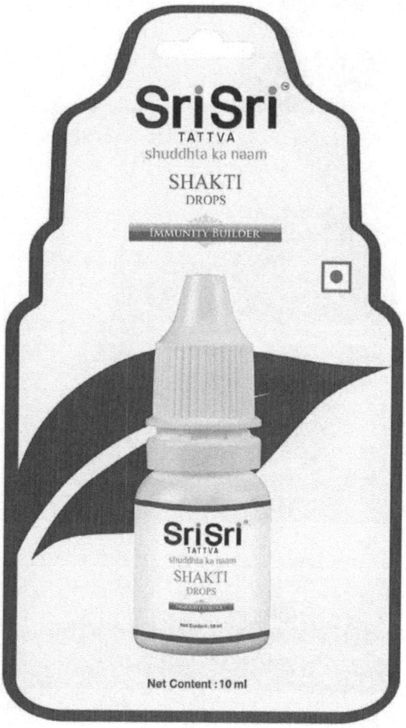

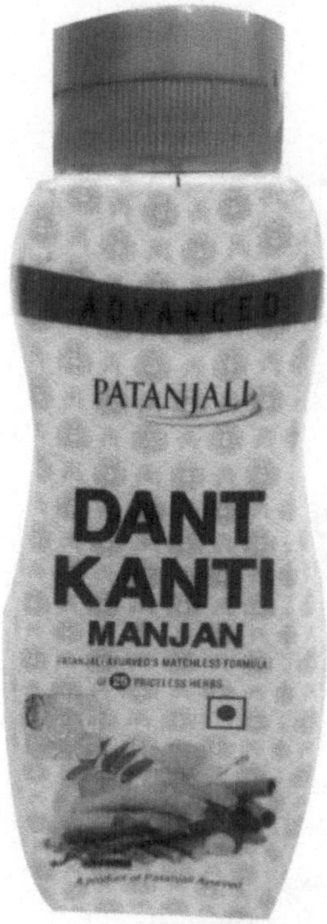

Keeping healthy teeth and gums is no longer possible by regular brushing alone due to a drastic intake of packaged and fast foods. Daily dant manjan is a must.

Complete Set of 12 Poses

12 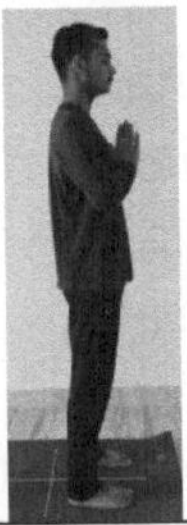		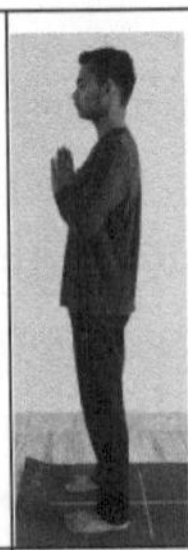 1 Namaste
11 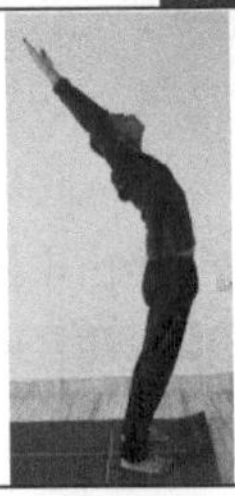		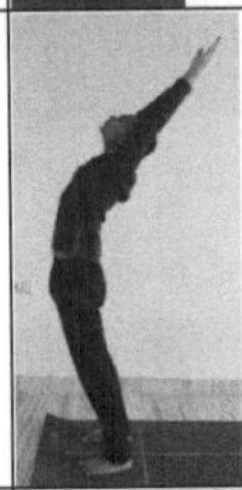 2
10 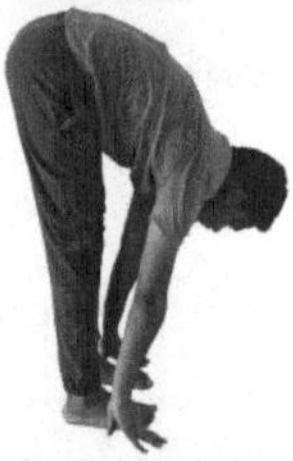		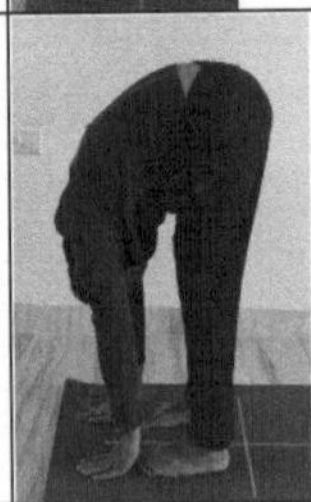 3
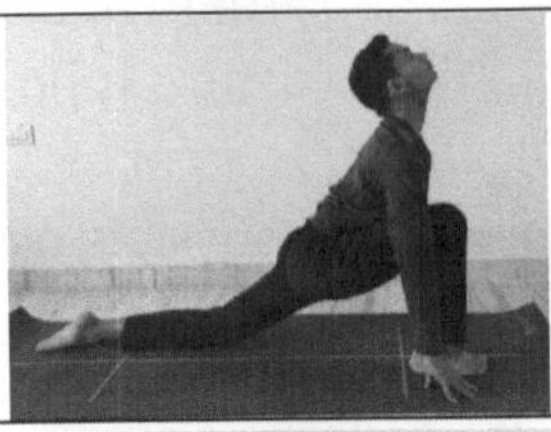 9		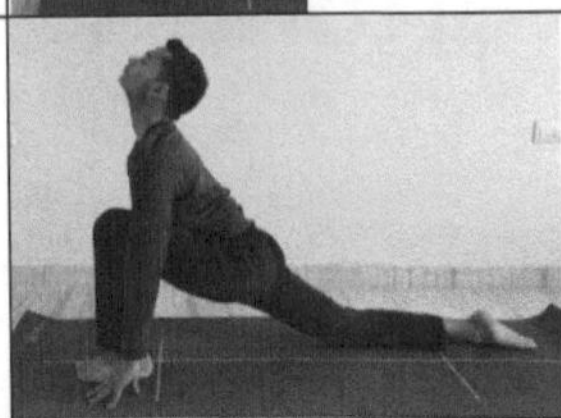 4
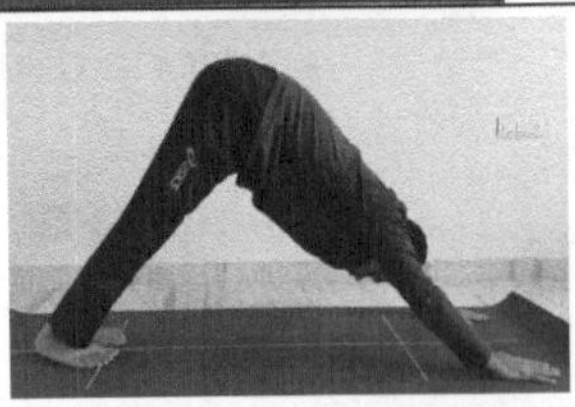 8		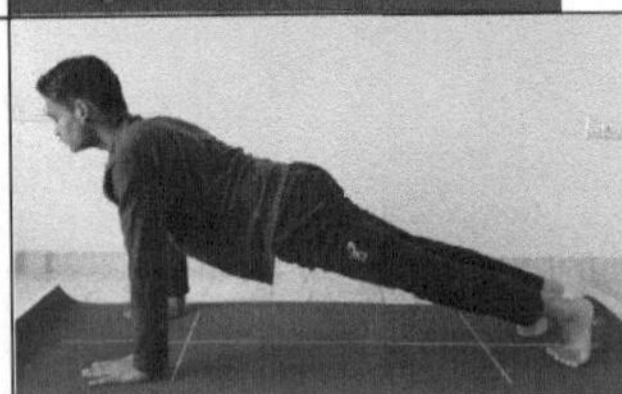 5
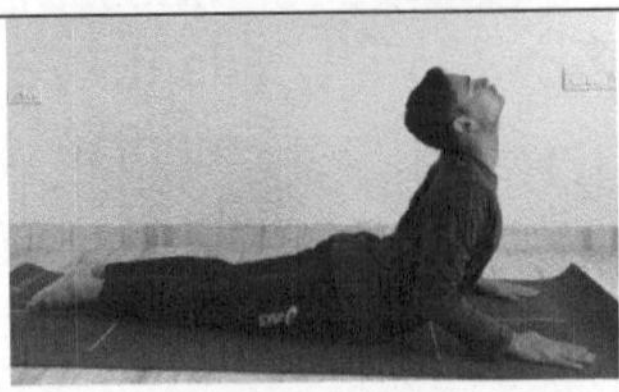 7		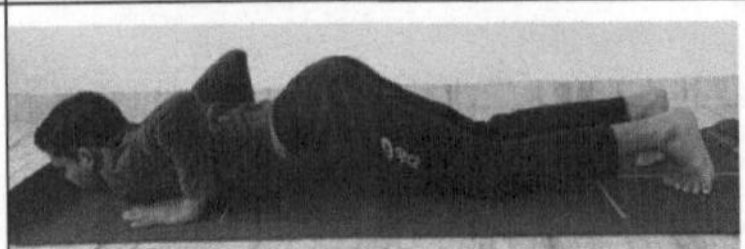 6

Alternate View of 12 Poses

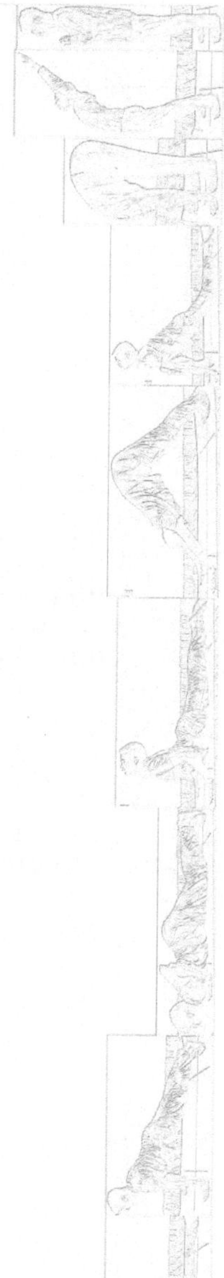

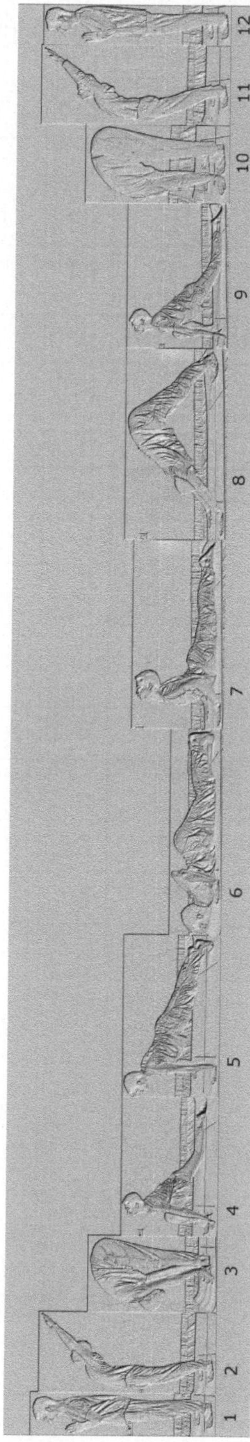

Latin Transliteration Chart

International Alphabet of Sanskrit Transliteration (I.A.S.T.)

a	ā	i	ī	u	ū	ṛ	ṝ	ḷ	
अ	आ	इ	ई	उ	ऊ	ऋ	ॠ	ऌ	
						◌ृ	◌ॄ	◌ॢ	
e	ai	o	au	ṃ	m̐	ḥ	Ardha Visarga	oṃ	
ए	ऐ	ओ	औ	◌ं	◌ँ	◌ः	ᳲ	ॐ	
Consonants are shown with a vowel 'a= अ' for uttering									
ka	क	ca	च	ṭa	ट	ta	त	pa	प
kha	ख	cha	छ	ṭha	ठ	tha	थ	pha	फ
ga	ग	ja	ज	ḍa	ड	da	द	ba	ब
gha	घ	jha	झ	ḍha	ढ	dha	ध	bha	भ
ṅa	ङ	ña	ञ	ṇa	ण	na	न	ma	म
ya	ra	la	va		ḷa	'			
य	र	ल	व		ळ	ऽ			
					Consonant only				
śa	ṣa	sa	ha		ka	क्अ = क			
श	ष	स	ह		k	क्			

References

https://www.ashtangayoga.info/philosophy/sanskrit-and-devanagari/transliteration-tool/

http://www.sarahburgessyoga.com/about-yoga/

https://srisrischoolofyoga.org/in/

Track - Surya Namaskar Mantra , Artist - Sahil Jagtiani
https://www.youtube.com/watch?v=fmusOSPHSxI

Sun Salutation, as per the Sivananda Yoga tradition
https://www.youtube.com/watch?v=bWJ2VBTt344

Surya Namaskar (Sun Salutations) | Art Of Living Yoga
https://www.youtube.com/watch?v=-o2QXWBPS3k

Sun Salutation by Brooklyn Yoga School founder, Lily Cushman
https://www.youtube.com/watch?v=73sjOu0g58M

Demonstrated by Shiva das
https://www.youtube.com/watch?v=mtO2fRmh8D8

Baba Ramdev
https://www.youtube.com/watch?v=76JRRnUfTI0

Surya Kriya - Fire Up The Sun Within | Isha Hatha Yoga
https://www.youtube.com/watch?v=_wq-OiPk-pU

Ashwini Kumar Aggarwal, Devotees of Sri Sri Ravi Shankar Ashram, Punjab, Publications.
– Bhagavad Gita Applied Wisdom – 1st – 2018.
– Patanjali Yoga Sutras: Essence and Sanskrit Grammar – 1st – 2018.
– Prashna Upanishad: Essence and Sanskrit Grammar – 1st – 2020.

Epilogue

The Sun is the undeniable source of energy and power on the entire planet. It is not just a physical factor, it is also the prime mover that awakens, guides, and stimulates the spirit. We receive so much from the Sun, can we do a bit in return?

YES we can. Surya Namaskar. Honoring the Sun. Accepting the bounty of the Sun with a grateful and humble countenance.

One may not believe it, nor may we prove it, but our honor reaches and touches the heart of the Sun. And makes it more benevolent.

सर्वे भवन्तु सुखिनः । सर्वे सन्तु निरामयाः ।
सर्वे भद्राणि पश्यन्तु । मा कश्चिद् दुःख भाग् भवेत् ॥
ॐ शान्तिः शान्तिः शान्तिः ॥

When faith has blossomed in life,
Every step is led by the Divine.

Sri Sri Ravi Shankar

Om Namah Shivaya

जय गुरुदेव

9 788194 733898

Printed at Repro India Ltd.